Dr Stuart Mason

The Dieting Handbook

Everything You Need to Know to Lose Weight Permanently

Table of Contents

Part One - Nutrition

Part Two - Diet Plans Examined

Part Three - Digging Deeper

Part Four - The Processed Food Industry

Part Five - Lose Weight Sensibly

Part One - Nutrition

What is it?

Nutrition is the name given to the process by which all living creatures absorb compounds essential for life. These compounds are known as nutrients and include fats, carbohydrates, proteins, minerals, vitamins and water. With them, we can generate the energy we need to function, regulate and repair ourselves.

However, for optimum health, our bodies need other things as well, one of the most important of which is fibre. This is found only in plants - meat and fish do not contain any.

Fibre is an essential part of a healthy, balanced diet and helps prevent heart disease, diabetes, weight gain and some cancers. It also improves digestive health. Another is calcium - this is a compound used to build and maintain bones

However, a nutritious diet is just one factor in achieving good health. It's also important that the energy created by nutrition, i.e. calories, is put to good use. If it isn't, two things happen:

The first is that the body stores the energy as fat in the anticipation that it may be needed at some other time - essentially, it's a backup. Exactly the same thing happens if you eat too much - the body has more energy than it can use and rather than just throw it away, it stores it in the form of fat for a rainy day.

Secondly, our bodies are controlled by muscles and without them we can do absolutely nothing. The more we use these muscles, the stronger and more efficient they become. This leads to increased physical strength, endurance and stamina. Our organs are controlled by muscles as well. For example, cardiac muscle in the heart is responsible for pumping blood around the body. The stronger all these muscles are, the greater the overall health of the body.

However, if we don't exercise to use the energy, the opposite happens. Our muscles become weak and so we are able to do less physically - everything becomes an effort. More dangerous, however, is the effect on our vital organs, such as the heart, lungs, liver and the kidneys. Weak, under-used muscles in any of these results in reduced functionality that make us feel unwell, restrict our ability to do basic things and, ultimately, are the cause of illness, disease and, all too often, premature death.

Our diets can also be affected by factors such as genetics, our environment, age and culture. Many people have to take these into account when deciding what they can and cannot eat. For example, there may be a family history of heart disease, or risk factors such as high blood pressure, that rule certain foods out. Young and active people need more food than older or less active ones. Also, people who are trying to lose weight can find it difficult to get the nutrients they need due to their necessarily restricted diet.

In this book, I show how to ensure you have a healthy, balanced diet that will keep your body firing on all cylinders. This will, without doubt, be the single most effective thing you can do, to not just feel good but also vastly reduce the likelihood of getting dangerous illnesses and diseases.

The ones I am talking about are cancer, heart disease, stroke, high blood pressure, diabetes and osteoporosis. Currently, these are all rife, particularly in the western hemisphere, and ruin millions of lives every year. Much of it is preventable and a healthy diet is the starting point.

Some pertinent quotes:

"Let food be your medicine, and medicine be your food" - Hippocrates

"He who has health has hope, and he who has hope has everything." - Arabian Proverb

Nutritional Status

Nutritional status is basically an assessment of a person's body from a dietary standpoint. Factors taken into account are what the person eats, the types of nutrient in their body and if there are enough of those nutrients to enable them to function efficiently.

More specifically, the assessment looks at the essential nutrients. These come in two classes:

1) Macronutrients - these are nutrients that generate the large amount of energy the body needs in order to grow and maintain itself. They are found in fats, protein and carbohydrates

2) Micronutrients - found in vitamins and minerals, these play a vital role in the body's general health and well-being

Other factors considered include appearance and the blood levels of various compounds. How a person looks will give a dietician a lot of information. For example, the condition of their skin, hair and nails offers clear clues as to how well nourished they are.

The presence of normal amounts of fat and muscle does as well. The dietician can also check that the person's weight is appropriate for their height, i.e. their body mass index (BMI).

A blood test is a more scientific method of assessing someone's nutritional status. It does this by showing what's in their blood and so, by extension, what's in their body. For example, a person who is malnourished will have low levels of certain proteins. A high level of cholesterol indicates a person may drink too much alcohol. A blood test can also highlight irregularities in body functions that need to be treated with an appropriate diet.

Factors such as access to food, existing chronic conditions and the ability to eat food are also indicators of nutritional status. As are certain medical conditions, such as Crohn's disease, that limit a person's ability to absorb nutrients from food they've eaten.

Sadly, despite the clear benefits of having their nutritional status assessed, very few people ever think to have it done. Indeed, many people have never even heard of it. In most cases, it's the fact they are putting on excess weight that eventually persuades them something is amiss.

However, if something is wrong internally, it won't be so obvious. For this reason, I suggest everyone should have their nutritional status checked periodically. Many people are shaken by the results.

Recognising Nutrient Deficiencies

It is a known fact that the vast majority of people have a diet that does not provide all the nutrients required for a long and healthy life. Given that in most parts of the world there is no shortage of food, this does seem perverse.

One reason for it is ignorance - many people just don't realise how important a balanced diet actually is. Other reasons are stupidity, laziness and lack of self-control. Many people are simply too idle, or too silly, to cook proper food. Instead, they rely on fried chicken and fish, pizzas and other types of processed food. Indeed, many people are quite happy to eat food that they know isn't good for them.

Even people who are aware of the importance of their diet, and take care to ensure they are eating healthily, still get caught out. One way this can happen is that they get a condition that affects their ability to absorb nutrients. Another common cause is the big processed food corporations. All too often, they sell us food that is not as rich in a particular nutrient as they would have us believe.

Luckily, most nutrient deficiencies eventually manifest themselves in one way or another - some you can see, some you can feel and some you can hear. The trick is spotting the signs, being able to interpret them and acting on them.

Lets take a look at the most common nutrient deficiencies:

Iron

About a quarter of the world's population is thought to be deficient in iron. This essential mineral is found in every cell in the body and is used to make oxygen-carrying proteins called haemoglobin and myoglobin.

When your iron level is too low, you become anaemic. This is a condition whereby the lack of iron in the body causes a reduction in the number of red blood cells. As these store and carry oxygen in the blood, having less of them than you should means your organs and tissues won't get as much oxygen as they need.

The most common symptoms are tiredness and lethargy, shortness of breath and heart palpitations. You may also experience headaches, tinnitus, loss of hair, impaired sense of taste and difficulty swallowing. Furthermore, it can make you more susceptible to illness and infection as it adversely affects your immune system.

Iron deficiency is not necessarily diet related. It can also be caused by stomach ulcers, stomach and bowel cancer and by taking non-steroidal anti-inflammatory drugs.

Good sources of iron include fish, eggs, leafy green vegetables, brown rice, beans, nuts, seeds, meat and dried fruit.

Iodine

A large proportion of the world's population is affected by iodine deficiency. This is a mineral that is essential for the production of thyroid hormones. These ensure the body's metabolic rate – the speed at which chemical reactions take place – are optimal.

The most common symptom is a swelling of the thyroid gland, which causes a lump to form in the front of the neck. Others include a dry mouth, dry skin, poor memory and concentration, an increase in heart rate and shortness of breath. Severe cases (with children in particular) can cause mental retardation and abnormal development.

One of the best ways to get iodine is to eat sea vegetables, such as kelp, nori, kombu and wakame. Other good sources are eggs, fish and dairy produce. You can also get small amounts of iodine from fruit and vegetables - this is largely dependent though on factors such as soil quality, the type of fertilizer used and the method of irrigation.

Vitamin D

Vitamin D is a fat-soluble vitamin that helps to regulate the amounts of calcium and phosphate in our bodies. These nutrients are required to keep our bones, teeth and muscles healthy. Deficiencies can cause bone deformities, such as rickets in children and a condition called osteomalacia (bone ache) in adults.

Symptoms that indicate a lack of vitamin D are depression, excessive head sweating, fatigue and general aches and pains. A deficiency in vitamin D is not usually obvious, however, as it often develops gradually, and thus unnoticed, over a period of time.

Unlike most vitamins that can only be acquired from the foods we eat, vitamin D is made by the body. So although some foods do contain small quantities of it, diet isn't really a factor. What *is* important is sunlight. Our bodies manufacture vitamin D from cholesterol in the skin when it is exposed to the sun. And as many people don't get enough exposure to the sun, they don't have enough vitamin D.

This is the best way to get it - fifteen minutes of sun twice a week is enough for most people. Foods such as oily fish, red meat, liver and eggs are the best dietary sources, albeit a poor second best. It is also possible to get vitamin D in the form of pill supplements.

Calcium

Calcium is a mineral that's essential for life. In addition to building teeth and bones, and maintaining them, it helps our blood clot, enables our nerves to send messages around the body and helps our muscles to contract and expand.

A diet deficient in calcium does not produce obvious symptoms in the short-term because the body maintains its calcium level by taking it from bone when supplies are low. Over the long-term, however, this weakens the bones and can result in osteoporosis and, with children, rickets. Both increase the likelihood of bone fractures.

A good source of calcium is unboned fish - one tin of sardines provides nearly 50 percent of the recommended daily amount. Others include dairy products and dark green leafy vegetables. Some people take calcium supplements but this really isn't necessary given that it's present in so many foods.

Magnesium

Magnesium is crucial to nerve transmission, muscle contraction, blood coagulation, energy production, nutrient metabolism and bone and cell formation. Nearly 50 percent of people are lacking in this essential nutrient.

As it plays such an important role in so many of the body's functions, a magnesium deficiency can have a large number of symptoms. These include difficulty sleeping, facial tics, cramps, eye twitching, migraines, loss of appetite, headaches and nausea. It can also be the cause of numbness, seizures, abnormal heart rhythms and personality changes.

The best source of magnesium is almonds - a handful of these nuts provides around fifteen percent of the recommended daily amount. Cashews and peanuts are not far behind. Also good are avocados, beans (black in particular), grains, potatoes, brown rice, yoghurt and leafy green vegetables - spinach especially.

You should also be aware that certain foods and drinks can deplete the level of magnesium in your body. Regular consumption of foods high in sugar - cakes, candy, biscuits, pastries, etc - causes the body to excrete magnesium via the kidneys.

Ditto caffeinated drinks like tea and coffee, carbonated drinks like soda and also alcohol. Certain drugs, including diuretics, heart and asthma medication, and birth control pills do the same.

Nutrition Myths

Nutrition research has come a long way in the last few years. Despite this, however, a lot of people still give credence to outdated theories and ideas. For example, that fat is bad for you, eating eggs raises cholesterol and that gluten should be avoided Many of these have come about due to simple misconceptions. Others are due to a deliberate policy of misinformation by food manufacturers. Then there's the Internet - the first port of call for many people when they decide to alter their diet. Unfortunately, a lot of what they read here is pure myth.

So before we go any further, I'll take a look at some of these myths and theories and see what the reality is. In no particular order, we have:

Fresh fruit & veg is healthier than frozen
Wrong - fresh fruit and vegetables are usually *less* healthy. This is due to a process known as respiration, whereby all fruits and vegetables continue to breathe after being harvested. This breaks down their fat, carbohydrate and protein content, which leads to loss of both flavour and nutrients. It also causes their sugar levels to go up.

However, when they are frozen, the respiration stops,

and the sugar and nutrients are preserved at the existing level - sugar low, nutrients high.

Gluten-free diets are healthier

No, they're not. Assuming you don't have an intolerance to gluten, or have Coeliac disease, there is absolutely no reason to remove gluten from your diet. Gluten is found in wheat, barley and rye, which means it's in many carb-based foods such as biscuits, pies, cakes and pastries. These are all foods you shouldn't be eating as we'll see later, but the presence of gluten is not the reason.

Saturated fat is bad for you

Most health authorities are still making this claim with regard to heart disease. However, recent studies have demonstrated that it's not true at all. In fact, not only is saturated fat actually good for you, it is absolutely essential. Consider this simple fact - human breast milk is 54 percent saturated fat. Would nature give babies saturated fat if it was bad for them? It is only bad when eaten in excessive quantities - something that applies to all foods!

Studies show that it's actually the trans fats made from vegetable oils, excessive carbohydrate intake, obesity, high blood pressure and sedentary lifestyles that are really behind the heart disease epidemic.

Egg yolks should be avoided

Eggs have been castigated for years because of the high level of cholesterol and saturated fat in the yolks. However, what the health agencies who propagate this nonsense don't tell you, or perhaps aren't even aware of, is that cholesterol is extremely beneficial to your health.

So much so, in fact, the liver actually makes it as very few people get enough through their diet. The more cholesterol you eat, the less has to be made by the liver, and vice versa. In other words, the body always keeps its cholesterol level in balance.

A very large recent study found no association between egg consumption and heart disease or stroke. Other, earlier, studies have reached the same conclusion. Quite clearly, the cholesterol and saturated fat content of eggs isn't an issue.

Carbohydrates are bad for you

This myth has been around for a while now, and is due to the popularity of low-carb diets such as the Atkins. The 'carbs are bad' theory from Dr Atkins and co has led to many people being confused about this foodstuff and its role in our health.

The answer is yes and no. It all depends on the type, quality and amount of carbohydrate being eaten.

Carbohydrates that are highly processed, such as those used in biscuits, cereals, breads, cakes, pasta, crackers and so on, have had most, if not all, of the nutrients refined out of them. These foods also have a very high sugar content, which is bad for people as it makes them put on excessive amounts of weight with the all attendant health issues this brings.

The carbohydrates that *are* good for you are the ones that have either not been processed at all, or just minimally. These do contain nutrients and include all vegetables, fruit, nuts, seeds and legumes.

Salt is bad for you
Not only is salt supposed to be bad for you in general, it can also contribute to cardiovascular disease apparently. However, years of scientific research has failed to show any evidence of this.

Salt is actually an essential nutrient - we simply cannot live without it. A diet too low in salt can give rise to a dangerous condition known as hyponatremia - when the level of sodium in the blood is abnormally low.

Essentially, there are two types of salt - natural salt as found in lakes and the seas, and table salt - highly processed and so far less healthy.

The latter is created by super-heating natural salt, the act of which destroys virtually all its nutrients. The salt is then bleached and cleaned with a chemical solution to make it pure white. Lastly, compounds such as moisture absorbents and anti-caking agents are added to make it easy to pour and sprinkle on food.

While table salt won't give you a stroke or heart attack, neither does it do you any good due to its lack of nutrients. Natural salt, however, does.

A calorie is a calorie is a calorie

It's not, far from it actually. The body stores and utilises calories in various ways that are dependant on the nutrients in the food. As an example, lets compare eating oats and eating fish. Oats contain a type of starch known as 'resistant starch' which is resistant to digestion. Fish, however, doesn't. As a result, the body is unable to absorb and use as many calories from the oats as it can from the fish.

It's a similar story with high-protein foods like poultry. Protein is a high-thermogenic food, which requires an expenditure of energy to digest, absorb and transport it's nutrients to the body's cells. Fats and carbohydrates, on the other hand, are low-thermogenic foods that don't require energy to be used.

Everything else being equal then, calories from fats and carbohydrates will make you gain more weight than an equivalent amount of calories from protein.

Brown bread is better for you than white bread
Indeed it is, assuming you can find some that is actually made with whole grain. Unfortunately, the vast majority of brown bread sold is simply white bread coloured with caramel or molasses to give the appearance of a brown loaf. Nutritionally, it will be no better.

To ensure you don't fall for this con, check the loaf's packaging for the words 'whole grain' or '100% whole wheat'. Also, the first ingredient listed should be a grain of some type, i.e. oats wheat, rye, barley, etc. If it is, you have the genuine article and it will indeed be healthier.

Dairy produce is unhealthy
Another myth perpetuated by the 'saturated fat is bad for you' brigade. Dairy products such as cheese and butter do contain high levels of saturated fat but, as we have already seen, it has now been established that saturated fats are actually very good for us.

Their fat content apart, dairy products are also full of essential nutrients such as protein, zinc, B vitamins and calcium. Furthermore, weight-loss diets that include dairy produce have been shown to be more effective than diets that omit them.

Organic produce is more nutritious
This one is true but only to a degree. The fact is, the nutritional difference between organically grown and conventionally grown produce is not that great. For most people, it is not enough to justify the expense of going organic. However, for people who take their health seriously, it is, although maybe only just.

It also has to be said that organic food is much less likely to be polluted with pesticides, and so may be worth the extra expense for this reason alone.

You need to drink eight glasses of water a day
Eight glasses is approximately two litres and, together with your water intake from the food you eat and other liquids, is far more than the average person needs. When you need water, your body will tell you - you will suddenly be thirsty - it's as simple as that.

This is a myth propagated by the bottled water industry. When you read this claim, you're reading a marketing stratagem - take no notice.

Eating at night will make you put on weight
Eating at night has long been associated with weight gain. However, the fact is, a calorie is a calorie, regardless of when you eat it. What does make you put on weight is eating more calories than you burn.

It doesn't matter what time of day you eat. It is what and how much you eat, and how much physical activity you do during the day, that determines whether you gain, lose or maintain weight.

Red wine is good for you
There is no question about this - red wine is indeed good for you as it has a high content of antioxidants, such as resveratrol. These fight free radicals (rogue cells that can cause enormous damage) and so reduce the risk of conditions like cancer and heart disease. What's not to like then?

Well, maybe the fact that red wine is, like all alcohol, actually a neurotoxin - a poison. It may be that the benefits of drinking small amounts (one small glass daily is the suggested limit) outweigh the poisonous effects on the brain. On the other hand, they may not!

As these benefits can also be had by simply eating less and exercising more, why take the risk? If the thought of not drinking alcohol at all bothers you, remember why you're reading this book!

Eat many small meals throughout the day
The theory behind this claim is that by eating more frequently than normal but eating less when you do, your metabolism will remain high. This stops you getting hungry and also controls your blood sugar level.

As a result, you eat less overall and so lose weight.

It's a nice theory but unfortunately it doesn't work in practice. It may raise your metabolism slightly but it's the amount of food eaten that controls hunger levels, not the number of meals. In fact, research has shown that eating many small meals a day actually makes people want to eat more - not less.

It should also be pointed out that it's unnatural for our bodies to be constantly in the fed state. In years gone by, it was the norm to go without food for long periods of time, i.e. fast. Research has shown that this is actually good for us.

Low-fat foods are good for you
For a long time now, the mantra has been that people concerned about their weight, or eating for a healthy heart, should eat low-fat foods. As a result, sales of high-fat foods such as dairy produce, have dropped.

In response, the manufacturers have removed much of the saturated fat from their products in an attempt to make them appear healthier. However, they have replaced the saturated fat with hydrogenated oil (trans fats). Furthermore, in order to make the low-fat food palatable (most of a food's flavour is in the fat), they have also had to add large amounts of sugar.

What's happened then, is that in these low-fat foods healthy saturated fats have been replaced with trans fats, refined carbohydrates and sugar - all of which are bad for us. So, they can in fact be positively dangerous.

Omega-6 is bad for you

Omega-6 is a polyunsaturated fat - one of a number of fatty acids found in certain foods and virtually all vegetable oils.

As to whether it is bad for you, the answer is both yes and no. Omega-6 actually provides many benefits - these include keeping blood pressure low, lowering the risk of heart disease, fighting inflammation, stimulating skin and hair growth, maintaining bone health and many others. It is, in fact, essential for good health.

The problems come when it is taken in excess, as it is in most western countries, due to it's prevalence in processed foods. All of a sudden, a fat that can be really good for us becomes the instigator of a number of health problems. These include heart disease, cancer, alzheimer's, rheumatoid arthritis, diabetes and many more.

The polyunsaturated fat most people should be eating a lot more of is omega-3. The ideal ratio of omega-3 to omega-6 fats is 1:1, but in the typical western diet it is between 1:20 and 1:50.

Vegetarian diets are healthier
A vegetarian (vegan) diet consists of nothing but plants and foods made from plants. Vegans don't eat anything that comes from animals.

The problem with this is that human beings are omnivores - we are designed to function at our best when eating plants *and* animals. A lot of important nutrients are omitted in a vegetarian diet. Vitamin B12 is one example - others are protein, vitamin D, iron, zinc and calcium.

There are no studies that show a vegan diet to be healthier than diets that include meat. If a person on a vegan diet is healthy, it's more likely to be because they are health-conscious generally, i.e. they exercise, don't smoke or drink, etc. Not eating meat is immaterial.

The lack of animal nutrients, vitamin B12 and protein in particular, actually makes the vegan diet less healthy. In fact, it can be positively dangerous for children.

All sugar should be avoided
Another word for sugar is energy. And as we all need energy to function, it follows that it can't be bad for us.

And indeed, in small amounts, it isn't. Sugar is only a problem when we eat too much of it - as most of us do!

This is because our livers can only deal with a small amount, currently thought to be about six teaspoons a day. Any more is converted into fat. The problem is exacerbated when we eat refined sugar, such as table sugar. With nothing to slow its absorption, the liver can be overwhelmed.

When you eat sugar in its natural form - in a piece of fruit for example - you are also eating fibre, minerals and vitamins - these reduce the rate at which the sugar is absorbed in the body and so ease the load on the liver. Plus, the fibre is satiating and stops you eating too much of the fruit and, hence, sugar.

A related issue is that sugar can be addictive. A large dose of refined sugar gives an instant high which is soon followed by a low - this creates an urge to eat more sugar. Do it too many times and you can end up being addicted to the stuff.

So remember, as long as you restrict your intake to no more than six teaspoons daily, eating sugar - either natural or refined - won't cause you any problems.

Metabolic Typing

Many people are trying to lose weight, improve their health generally or improve it in a specific way; and there's many people offering them advice on how to do it. Sometimes the advice works but as often as not it doesn't - indeed, in many cases, it has been known to make things worse.

Government health agencies are also at it. For years now, they have been advocating a diet low in fat and high in carbs. Supposedly, this will make us lose weight while, at the same time, improve our cardiovascular health. However, what's actually happened is an obesity crisis the like of which has never been seen before. Even worse, the knock-on is a diabetes epidemic that has blighted millions of lives around the world. All-in-all, it has been an unmitigated disaster.

Then there are all the diet plans - the 5:2 diet, the Dukan diet, the Paleo diet, the Atkins diet and the Cambridge diet to mention just some. They are all different but claim to do the same thing - help you to lose weight and become more healthy. However, the reality is that while these diets do help some people, they don't help others.

Nuts provide numerous health benefits for most people but cause headaches and digestive issues for others. Garlic may be a superfood but can also be the villain behind gallbladder pain. A person with hypoglycemia will have different dietary needs than someone with type 2 diabetes and an athlete will have different needs than someone who is less active.

The point I am making here is that there is no such thing as an ideal diet that works for everyone. If that is what you are seeking, you are extremely unlikely to find it. For optimum results, you need a customised diet plan that will take into account factors such as taste preferences, genetics, ethnicity, age and general health. This is individualized nutrition and is what's meant by the term metabolic typing.

Now, in theory, you can do this yourself. It will, however, be a frustrating process as the only way you'll be able to do it is through trial and error - try something for a while and see if it works. If it doesn't, try something else. An approach like this can take a very long time and it's quite probable you'll lose interest after a while and simply stop bothering.

Another option is to take an online Metabolic Type test. Take my advice and give these a wide berth - they'll want your life history before you are allowed anywhere near the test and then, at the end, you will be given a 'chance' to buy some product they are flogging off. Don't waste your time. The best approach by far is to get a nutrition expert to do it for you. The following will explain why:

A friend of mine, Andy Robins, began having digestive issues (he declined to specify what, exactly!). Apart from being slightly overweight, he considered himself to be in good shape - he was active, had a varied diet and had many interests in life. After putting up with it for a while, he decided to visit his doctor and was advised to see a nutrition specialist.

So Andy booked an appointment in a health clinic where he was given a Metabolic Type test. The first part of this involved keeping a diary of everything he ate and drank, and at what times. He also had to record what exercise he took and when, when he slept and for how long, precise details of his bowel movements - size, shape, colour, etc, and how he felt generally at various times of the day. This went on for two weeks.

After analysing the results of the test, Andy was told that his problem was being caused by an over-consumption of grain-based products - bread, tortillas and cereal, specifically. The suggested cure was to cut down on the amount of these he ate and, rather than have cereal for breakfast, have a smoothie. This was to consist of a dark green vegetable, such as kale, a lemon, coconut, blueberries, protein powder and a handful of mixed nuts. He was also told his fat level was too low and advised to eat more foods rich in saturated fat like cheese and meat.

Within days, literally, Andy's digestive issue had cleared up. This wasn't all though - it was also pointed out to him that he wasn't getting enough sleep due to a tendency to wake up in the early hours for sometimes long periods. The specialist explained that a common cause of this is irregularity in blood sugar levels. When it is low, the body responds with a shot of adrenalin, which can be enough to wake some people.

He was told to eat a banana for a carb boost just before turning in for the night. Surprise, surprise - it worked. Andy's sleep improved and he felt a lot better for it. He also found he was less hungry and so began eating less with the result he soon lost the few pounds he was overweight by. When he went back to see the specialist, he was told this was because lack of sleep increases appetite and decreases satiety.

The reason you are reading this book is that you want to get yourself in shape. Good health is an incredibly important issue and you must be prepared to do whatever it takes to achieve it.

The first step is to start eating the foods, and only the foods, that will fuel your body to the maximum extent. You also want to eat foods that are good for you in specific ways, as Andy now is.

The best way to ensure that you do is to get a Metabolic Type test done. As a bonus, the test may also highlight health issues of which you weren't aware.

So, I highly recommend that you go out and book one now!

The Low-down on Fat

The subject of dietary fat is very confusing to many people. Some experts say fat is good for us while other experts say the opposite. Some say we need a certain amount of one type of fat and less of another. What's the truth though? Who do you believe?

Well, to start with, it's an indisputable fact that fat is an absolutely essential part of out diets. It provides our bodies with energy and supports cell growth. It helps protect our organs, keeps our skin and hair healthy, and stops us getting cold by placing a layer of insulation directly under the skin. Fat helps us absorb nutrients and much of a food's flavour comes from the fat it contains.

However, it comes in several types and it's this fact that causes much of the confusion. To get the benefits mentioned above, we need to eat the right types and in the right proportions. Get either, or both, wrong and it can actually be extremely bad for us.

The five main types of fat are:

- Saturated fat
- Polyunsaturated fat
- Monounsaturated fat
- Omega-3 fats

- Trans fats

These all have different chemical structures and physical properties. Lets take a look at each in more detail:

Saturated Fat
This is a type of fat that has two main sources. One is red meat - lamb and beef in particular. The other is vegetable oils - of these, palm oil, palm kernel oil and coconut oil contain the most. In fact, coconut oil is nearly 90 percent saturated fat.

For many years now, the medical establishment has been telling us that saturated fat, especially from animals, raises the level of cholesterol in our blood. This, supposedly, increases our risk of getting cardiovascular disease. However, despite fierce resistance from these people, the current line of thinking is that this theory has been wrong right from the start.

The truth of this is indicated by the fact that levels of heart disease and stroke have continued to rise despite food companies reducing the amount of saturated fat in their products.

In reality, saturated fat has been the fall guy for many years. It is, actually, very good for us but only when eaten in *sensible* quantities. Overdo it and you're in trouble - no question. Don't eat enough though, and you miss out on a wide range of nutrients that are vital for your health and well-being. The key, as with most things in life, is finding the right balance.

Polyunsaturated Fats

This type of fat is found mostly in plant-based foods and oils, such as safflower oil, corn oil, sunflower oil, flaxseeds and nuts (especially walnuts). Plants apart, the best source is fatty fish, e.g. salmon, trout, sardines, mackerel and herring.

Polyunsaturated fats provide a wide range of nutrients that help to develop and maintain the body's cells. Vitamin E for example - an antioxidant vitamin that many of us don't get nearly enough of. They are also necessary for blood clotting and muscle movement.

Monounsaturated Fats

Monounsaturated fats are found in a variety of foods and oils. The latter include peanut, canola, sunflower and sesame oil. Another good source is nuts and seeds of all types. Yet another is olives and avocados.

The major benefit of eating these fats is that they are good for cardiovascular health, thanks to the protection they offer against metabolic syndrome - a term that covers a range of related disorders, such as high blood pressure and high blood sugar.

Monounsaturated fats are also effective against insulin resistance, bone weakness, many cancers and mood issues such as depression.

Omega-3 Fats
Omega-3 fats are a type of polyunsaturated fat commonly found in foods such as oily fish, nuts and seeds, plant-based oils and beans.

They're thought to be beneficial for a whole range of conditions that include alzheimer's, macular degeneration, inflammation, diabetes and more. Because of this, omega-3 fats are all the rage, currently, and the food companies are taking advantage by adding them to their products.

However, all is not as it seems - as ever, the food companies are being less than honest. To understand why, you need to know that there are actually three types of omega-3 fats:

- DHA (Docosahexaenoic Acid)
- EPA (Eicosapentaenoic Acid)
- ALA (Alpha-Linolenic Acid)

The main source of DHA and EPA is oily fish, and it is these two omega-3 fats that confer the health benefits. ALA is sourced from plants and is far less effective. However, as it is much cheaper, it is ALA that the food companies add to their products and advertise for its 'amazing health benefits'. Once again, a complete con!

Trans Fats

Trans fats are made from vegetable oils in an industrial process known as hydrogenation. This involves adding hydrogen to vegetable oil, which causes the oil to become solid at room temperature. The benefit it offers the food companies is that it doesn't go off as quickly as natural oil does. As a result, foods made with it have a much longer shelf life.

Just one of the problems with these trans fats is that they cause calcification in our veins and arteries. This narrows them, thus decreasing the space available for blood to flow. If an affected person then has a blood clot, particularly in one of the coronary arteries, a stroke, or even death, can be the result.

Furthermore, studies have shown that trans fat consumption can also cause Alzheimer's disease, prostate and breast cancer, type 2 diabetes, liver dysfunction, infertility and depression.

Trans fats are found in all types of processed food. These include baked goods (pies, bread, cakes, biscuits, muffins), snacks (popcorn, chocolate, crisps), fried food (fish and chips, doughnuts, chicken). It is also a main ingredient in margarine.

Summary

Limited amounts of saturated fat, animal or vegetable, are very good for us, if not essential. Polyunsaturated and monounsaturated fats are also good for us and can be eaten more freely than saturated fat. Just remember they are fats and, as such, are fattening.

Trans fats are a different story altogether and should be avoided like the plague. This means you should stop eating *all* processed foods as of now! While it is true the food companies are beginning to reduce the amount of trans fats in their products, their use is still widespread and will be for some time to come.

What's The Deal With Cholesterol?

As with saturated fat, cholesterol has been vilified for years by the medical establishment. They would have you believe it is one of the major causes of heart disease. This theory has been supported by the big drug companies who produce cholesterol-lowering drugs. Does this suggest anything to you?

What is it though? Well, cholesterol is a waxy substance known as a lipid, and it is absolutely crucial for the normal functioning of the body. Most of it is made by the liver, but it is also present in some foods. The substance attaches itself to proteins in the blood, which carries it around the body.

A current theory is that there are two types of cholesterol - low-density lipoproteins (LDL) and high-density lipoproteins (HDL). One is supposed to be 'good' while the other is 'bad'. LDL is thought to be the latter as it creates a layer of plaque on the inside of the arteries. If this layer gets too thick, it can restrict the flow of blood and so eventually cause heart disease or stroke. HDL, on the other hand, is supposed to be good due to the fact it removes LDL cholesterol from the blood. That's the theory, at any rate!

The reality, however, is that there is no 'good' or 'bad' cholesterol - it's all one and the same. The lipoproteins are just tiny particles whose purpose is to carry essential fats in the blood around the body. In themselves, they are insignificant.

I've mentioned how crucial cholesterol is to the functioning of the body. Well, this is something of an understatement! It is actually essential at the cellular level - without it, there is no brain function, bone structure, muscles, reproductive system, memory or hormones - just nothing. Far from worrying about having too much of it, you should be concerned that you don't have enough!

The real villain, the one cholesterol has been taking the rap for all these years, is actually inflammation. This is a protective process that swings into action whenever there is a perceived threat to the body.

Cut your finger, for example, and several things happen immediately. Your blood will thicken, and maybe even clot, thus minimising blood loss; your immune system is activated in order to fight any potential infection; and your body manufactures new cells and sends them to the damaged area to effect repairs.

Now, in order to make these new cells, the body will need a dose of cholesterol so it sends a signal to the liver telling it to produce some. Once produced, the cholesterol is duly released into your blood.

Any damage that occurs internally triggers the same responses. And this is where we begin to see how cholesterol has been made the fall guy. As with the cut finger scenario, the body's response to internal damage is to thicken the blood, or even clot it. If this happens with a person who has restricted arteries, it will raise their blood pressure and, if one of these arteries is restricted enough to prevent the normal flow of blood, it will cause a heart attack or a stroke.

The cholesterol itself has nothing to do with it - all it does is to assist in the healing process. The heart attack/stroke is actually the result of inflammation somewhere in the body. As to what causes that inflammation, there are many things that could be responsible. It is, however, more than likely to be the result of a generally unhealthy lifestyle.

Now lets look at someone who goes to see a doctor about something. If their condition, whatever it is, is causing inflammation, the level of cholesterol in their blood will be raised. The doctor does a blood test to find out the cause of the condition and, noting the raised level of cholesterol, concludes they could be at risk of cardiovascular disease. So the person is put on a course of drugs to lower their cholesterol level.

While this will have absolutely no effect on the non-existent cardiovascular disease, it may well have an effect on the person's brain. It's a fact that people with very low cholesterol levels are more likely to be depressives. Typical symptoms are difficulty making a decision, confusion and agitation. It can even adversely affect sleeping patterns.

Then we have the cholesterol drugs themselves. These are a class of drug called statins and they reduce cholesterol by inhibiting an enzyme in the liver that produces it. However, they have effects other than the needless reduction of cholesterol.

For one, they can cause type 2 diabetes by raising the level of sugar in the blood. Muscle pain, damage to the liver, loss of memory and depression can also be caused by statins. These are drugs that you do not want to be taking unless there is absolutely no alternative!

The message, therefore, is clear. Cardiovascular disease has nothing to do with cholesterol. The main cause is restricted arteries due to eating the wrong foods (carbohydrates, sugar and trans fats). Overcooked food, lack of exercise, alcohol and smoking are other contributory factors.

Cut this rubbish out of your diet and replace it with proper foods, such as red meat, fish, eggs, vegetables and dairy produce. You should also have a good intake of healthy plant fats, such as coconut oil, olive oil, nuts, seeds and avocados.

Augment this much healthier diet with exercise. This needn't be too strenuous - a brisk twenty minute walk every day is all you need and will work wonders. Not only will it help you to lose weight, it will improve your circulation and boost the supply of oxygen to every cell in your body. Being fit will also help you to fight off diseases and illnesses as and when they manifest themselves.

The effects of exercise are not just physical either. A brisk walk is just as effective as anti-depressant pills in mild to moderate cases of depression. It makes the body release feel-good endorphins while, at the same time, reducing stress and anxiety. So put the pills back in the drawer and give it a try - it really does work!

How Nutrition Influences Cancer

The incidence of cancer globally has increased in just nine years from 13 million in 2008 to 15 million in 2017. Over the next twenty years, it is expected to hit 25 million a year.

These are frightening figures and are consistent with the equally frightening rise in obesity that is currently taking place. Are the two linked? The answer is yes, without doubt. Many studies have looked at the association between obesity and cancer and the results are quite conclusive - our weight has a major influence on whether or not we get cancer.

However, it's not just about weight. The types of food we eat are also a factor. Let's take a closer look, starting with the former:

Obesity

An excess of fat causes our bodies to produce proteins and hormones that adversely influence the way our cells work - this is a known cause of a number of diseases, just one of which is cancer.

It's thought that about 20 percent of cancers can be attributed to obesity. This is a quite startling figure and should be enough to make anyone who is overweight sit up and pay serious attention.

The types of cancer caused by obesity include cancers of the gallbladder, breast, bowel, womb, kidney, liver, oesophagus, stomach, pancreas and thyroid. Of these, breast and bowel cancer are most common, while pancreatic, oesophageal and gallbladder cancer are among the most difficult to treat.

Obesity is also known to affect the body's levels of sex hormones - oestrogen in particular. It affects insulin as well - the body's production of this increases in proportion to the amount of excess fat it is carrying. As hormones can cause body cells to grow and multiply, a surfeit of certain types of them can cause cancer. This is especially the case with breast cancer.

All-in-all, obesity is the second biggest cause of cancer after smoking.

Meat
The type of meat we are talking about here is red meat - lamb, beef and pork; and processed meat - bacon, sausages, hot dogs, salami, corned beef, beef jerky, ham and tinned meat.

While there is no definitive proof that eating meat causes cancer, it is thought to be possible when people eat abnormal amounts of it. For example, eat a twelve ounce steak every night for a number of years and you may well end up with bowel cancer. A more likely cause though, is cooking it at high temperatures, as when grilling or barbecuing. This is known to create dangerous chemicals that can cause cancer.

There is no evidence to suggest that white meat - chicken and fish - increases the risk of getting cancer.

The situation is different with processed meats. The World Health Organization (WHO) states quite clearly that they do cause cancer. A recent report said 50 grams of processed meat a day - less than two slices of bacon - increases the chance of developing colorectal cancer by 18 percent.

The cause is the chemicals used to process and preserve the meats. Two such are nitrites and nitrates, which act as preservatives by helping to prevent the growth of harmful bacteria. They also add a salty flavour, and improve the look of the meat products by giving them a red or pink colour. It is thought the body converts nitrites into cancer-causing chemicals called N-nitroso compounds.

However, as with red meat, the danger of eating processed meat has to be kept in proportion. The occasional bacon sandwich or hot dog is not going to hurt you at all - eat them every day though and they may well do!

Alcohol

An integral part of a person's diet is the liquid they drink. And many people drink a lot of alcohol. And the more alcohol they drink, the greater their risk of getting cancer. There is no debate about this - it's fact. These are, typically, cancers of the mouth, throat, breast, bowel, oesophagus, larynx and liver.

When you drink alcohol, your body converts it into a chemical called acetaldehyde. This can cause cancer by damaging DNA and preventing your body repairing the damage.

Furthermore, alcohol makes the body produce excess amounts of certain hormones. These tell the body's cells when to divide, amongst other things, and so increase the chances of cancer developing.

Yet another way alcohol can cause cancer is by damaging cells in the liver. Too much damage here results in a disease known as Cirrhosis, which increases the likelihood of developing cancer of the liver.

Note that drinking alcohol *and* smoking vastly increases the chances of getting cancer. This is because alcohol helps tissues in the mouth and throat to absorb the cancer-causing compounds found in tobacco smoke.

The message should be clear then. If you want to minimise the chances of getting cancer, your intake of alcohol must be very low. Actually, I recommend you cut it out of your life completely. It may be a short one if you don't!

Foods That Reduce the Risk of Cancer

Eating foods rich in fibre is known to reduce the risk of getting bowel cancer. One of the ways fibre does this is by helping the passage of food through our bowels. The quicker it happens, the less time the inner lining of the bowel is in contact with any harmful chemicals in the food. For example, chemicals such as those released when you consume alcohol and processed meats.

As a result, there's less chance of them being able to cause damage that could lead to cancer. Studies have shown that at least 10 percent of bowel cancer cases are linked to a diet low in fibre. This is one good reason to eat plenty of fruit and vegetables. Not only are they rich in fibre, they contain a variety of nutrients that help prevent many different types of cancers developing - mouth, throat and lung cancer in particular.

Physical activity has a preventative effect on cancer as well. Being active helps control levels of inflammation in the bowel which, if allowed to, can be the cause of cellular damage that leads to cancer.

Part Two - Diet Plans Examined

Those of you who have followed my advice and had your nutritional status checked out, and maybe even had a Metabolic Type test done, now have a good idea of what your diet needs to consist. Those of you who haven't, however, now have a decision to make - you can try the diet I recommend on pages 190-300 or buy a diet book - there's many to choose from.

Despite it being absolutely the best thing you can do, I know very few of you are going to take a Metabolic Type test, and for a number of reasons. They cost money, you may be too embarrassed to discuss your personal habits with a total stranger or there may not be a nutrition specialist near where you live.

So you are probably going to go for the second option - an existing diet plan. If so, and to help you choose the plan best suited to you, I am now going to take an unbiased look at the pros and cons of the most popular ones.

Atkins Diet
The Atkins is a low-carb, high-protein, eating plan created in 1972 by cardiologist Robert Atkins. The premise is that you begin with a low-carb diet for the first two weeks, during which time you are restricted to eating meat, seafood, eggs, cheese and specific

vegetables.

This first phase produces rapid weight loss that can be as high as 15lb. This is followed by three more phases during which you start eating increasing quantities of carbohydrates, fruit and vegetables. These subsequent phases will see a gradual reduction in the amount of weight lost. The diet also emphasises the importance of exercise.

Pros: the plan works - many people have lost weight with it. It's also good if you need to lose weight quickly for whatever reason.

The diet eliminates the refined carbohydrates found in foods such as white bread, cakes, pasta, biscuits, etc; and instead promotes unrefined carbs that are much healthier. It allows foods that other diets restrict - steak, bacon and eggs for example. This makes it easier to follow.

Cons: the amount of carbohydrate, and hence fibre, allowed on the diet is too low. This can cause a number of health issues such as nausea, headaches, weakness, dizziness, insomnia and constipation.

A large proportion of people who lose weight with the Atkins Diet, regain it once they've gone back to eating normally.

The diet does not contain sufficient minerals and vitamins, so supplementation is required to prevent nutritional deficiency.

Conclusion: while weight is lost initially, in the long term, it is difficult to sustain. This is due to the lack of carbohydrates - most people can only stick this for so long before going back to eating them. Furthermore, the rate at which weight is lost is usually too rapid to be healthy.

Over the long term, the diet can cause serious complications such as kidney disease, kidney stones, brittle bones and heart disease.

Dukan Diet

Similar to Atkins, the Dukan is a low-carb, high-protein diet. However, unlike Atkins, it restricts fat and omits vegetables completely in the first phase. These are gradually introduced in the subsequent phases of the diet.

The first 'attack' phase lasts for up to ten days and restricts you to a choice of 68 high-protein foods - no carbohydrates are allowed at all. The next 'cruise' phase allows you to start eating carbs as well as protein - you can choose from 28 approved vegetables. The third 'consolidation' phase adds fruit and dairy foods, and the fourth 'stabilisation' phase is basically a set of rules for life that stop you putting the weight back on.

Pros: initially, you can expect to lose weight quickly. The diet will appeal to those who don't want to spend their time counting calories and wondering if one food is better than another. Basically, it simplifies things by specifying just what you can and cannot eat.

Cons: the low carb and fibre intake causes the same problems as the Atkins diet.

In the long-term (and it is touted as being for life!), the diet can cause problems ranging from cancer and heart attack to premature aging. These are due to its nutritional deficiencies and lack of antioxidants.

Conclusion: firstly, the diet is not sustainable in the long term so most people regain the weight they've lost. More importantly, though, it is nutritionally unbalanced as it minimises the importance of fruit and vegetables, whole-grains and fibre. Not to mention the general health benefits of eating a variety of food types. This diet does your health no good at all.

5:2 Diet

This is, essentially, a part-time diet that allows you to eat normally five days of the week but for two non-consecutive days eat just a quarter of what you normally would. For women, this should be no more than 500 calories and, for men, 600 calories. On the 'eat' days, you can eat whatever you want. You can expect to lose approximately 1lb a week.

The diet employs the principle of intermittent fasting which not only helps in weight loss but can have other health benefits, such as reducing insulin resistance, suppressing inflammation and fighting free radical damage.

Pros: Weight is lost at a sensible, sustainable rate unlike with most diets. Also, you only have to count calories and feel hungry for two out of seven days. For many people, this makes it much easier to persevere with.

Cons: Quite a few. One major drawback is that people feel so deprived during the two fasting days that they overeat during the non-fasting days. As a result, they either lose no weight at all or actually put weight on!

Another is that the very low nutrient intake on fasting days can cause irritability, tiredness, lack of concentration and sleep issues. Also, exercise will be difficult on fasting days due to the low energy intake.

The diet can also have an impact on your social life - dinner and/or drinks with friends and family on fasting days will be a non-starter.

Conclusion: For many people, the diet works well

enough. However, the strict fasting aspect means it is unsuitable for people sensitive to drops in blood sugar levels, people with a history of eating disorders and people with type 1 diabetes.

Paleo Diet

The Paleo diet basically takes you back to the days of cavemen by restricting you to eating the foods they did. This is in the belief they were healthier than we are. Accordingly, you can only eat foods that can be hunted and fished - meat and seafood - and foods that can be collected - nuts, seeds, vegetables, fruits, herbs, spices and eggs.

Essentially, it is a low-carb, high-protein diet that eliminates grains, dairy produce, potatoes, refined sugar and salt. Healthy fats and oils like olive, flax and coconut are encouraged.

Pros: the Paleo diet lowers blood sugar levels and so is good for people suffering from type 2 diabetes. Also, the diet is 'cleaner' than most, given that the foods it permits have lower levels of additives and preservatives. Another plus is that it gives people a feeling of satiety due to the high amount of fats and protein.

Cons: the Paleo diet disregards the benefits provided by whole-grains. Not being able to eat dairy produce can mean an inadequate intake of some minerals - calcium being an important example. Also, for some people, the amount of protein in the diet may be too high.

Conclusion: it's a nice theory but does have some inherent flaws. Firstly, the idea that early humans didn't eat grain-based foods doesn't stand up to scrutiny. There is actually plenty of evidence that they were eating grasses, cereals, beans and legumes before the Paleolithic era even began.

Secondly, the diet assumes they were the same as we are today, and lived their lives in similar fashion. This is complete rubbish - for one, they were far more active than ever we are, which simple fact alone goes a long way to explaining their better health (assuming it was better!).

Having said all this, it is a diet that, with a bit of tweaking, i.e. including some grain-based foods, can be a very healthy one.

Alkaline Diet
The alkaline diet is touted as being able to help you not just lose weight but to also avoid issues such as osteoporosis, kidney and gall stones, cancer, arthritis and diabetes.

It works on the theory that dairy produce, eggs, meat, grains and processed foods produce an acidic waste product that adversely affects our body's pH (acidity and alkalinity) level. As a result, the likelihood of us getting the above-mentioned diseases is increased.

The diet supposedly works by cutting out the foods that do this and, instead, eating foods that have an alkaline-promoting effect on our bodies. The latter includes fruit, vegetables, nuts, seeds and legumes.

Pros: the only real advantage of this diet is that it makes you stop eating processed foods that are high in refined sugars and additives.

Cons: the first point that must be made here is that acid-forming foods aren't necessarily bad for us - in fact, most of them are actually highly nutritious. Even if they do have adverse effects, these are more than outweighed by the health benefits they offer.

Secondly, the idea that we can manipulate the body's pH level though diet is fantasy - our bodies regulate this themselves regardless of what we do or don't eat, Thirdly, it can actually damage our health by cutting out foods that are good for us.

Conclusion: this diet is highly endorsed by Hollywood celebrities and the like, which is probably reason enough to ignore it. It pretends to have a scientific basis (pH levels, etc) but there is no serious study that gives it credence. I suggest you give this one a wide berth.

Mediterranean Diet

One of the most well known diet plans of all is the Mediterranean diet. The basis of this plan is to eat the foods traditionally eaten in countries such as Italy and Greece. The inhabitants of these countries tend be healthier overall than those of other western nations. What's more, they have a much lower risk of getting serious diseases such as cancer, heart disease and type 2 diabetes.

The diet allows you to eat as much as you like of these foods: vegetables, seafood, potatoes, fruits, nuts, seeds, legumes, unrefined grains, herbs, spices, and healthy oils such as olive and coconut. Poultry, eggs and dairy produce can be eaten in moderation, while red meat is eaten rarely - maybe once a week.

Foods that cannot be eaten at all are basically anything that is highly processed.

With most diets, water, unsweetened tea and coffee are the only liquids that should be drunk. On the Mediterranean diet, however, you are also allowed one glass of red wine a day.

Pros: the 'diet' is not actually a diet - it's just a healthy way of eating that has evolved over many years. Most overweight people who try it naturally lose weight, albeit much more slowly than with regular diets as it is low in processed foods.

With regard to its fat content, this is largely of the monounsaturated type, which considerably lowers the risk of heart disease, many cancers, Alzheimer's disease and diabetes.

Cons: the amount of dairy produce that can be eaten is limited. This can result in a less than ideal intake of certain minerals, such as calcium. Another drawback is it can be a confusing diet to follow as specified parameters are vague, i.e. 'moderate', 'often', etc. So if you're the type of person who needs hard and fast rules to follow, this may not be the diet for you.

Conclusion: the Mediterranean diet is actually more of a lifestyle plan than a method of losing weight. It's a way of eating and drinking that, if followed for life, will result in a longer and healthier life than the average westerner achieves.

The Ketogenic Diet
The ketogenic diet is very low in carbs and very high in fats, and is similar to the Atkins and Dukan (both of which can sometimes end up being ketogenic if taken to extremes). The main difference is the amount of protein allowed - less with the ketogenic diet.

Following the diet will put you into ketosis. This is a condition that compels the body to produce tiny fuel molecules called ketones that it uses as an alternative fuel when blood sugar is in short supply (as it will be due to the very low level of carbohydrates).

As these ketones are produced from fat by the liver, the body turns into a fat-burning machine rather than the carbohydrate-burning machine it is normally. The reason protein is limited is that in the absence of carbohydrates, the body will turn it into sugar and so stay out of ketosis.

Pros: turning your body into a fat-burning machine is the ideal mechanism for weight loss. Furthermore, when in ketosis it produces much less of the fat-storing hormone, insulin. This can be extremely beneficial for people with type 2 diabetes.

Another benefit is that ketosis creates a steady flow of fuel to the brain - this is known to improve cognition and concentration. Many people use ketogenic diets specifically for this reason. Ketogenic diets are also a very effective treatment for people with epilepsy and have been used for this purpose for many years.

As if all that's not enough, a ketogenic diet has another trick up its sleeve - it can increase your level of physical endurance. This is because your body is being fuelled by its fat reserves which last much longer than stored carbohydrates that, typically, only last for an hour or two.

Having said that, there is evidence that suggests the *level* of performance achieved with ketosis is not as high as it is when you are fuelled by carbohydrates. You may be able to keep going longer but you won't be going as fast.

Cons: given the above, what's not to like as the saying goes? Well, it has to be said all is not rosy in the ketosis garden. For a start, it can take an adaptation period of up to two weeks to actually get into ketosis. During this period, you may feel rather grotty.

Also, those who need to expend high levels of energy - sportsmen and people doing manual labour, for example, may not be able to produce the amount of energy their particular activity requires while in ketosis.

By necessity (you have to eat *something* after all), your fat intake will be at a level that's high enough to maybe be detrimental to your health. Also, due to the highly restrictive nutritional guidelines - four grams of fat for every gram of protein or carbohydrate, it can be difficult to adhere to the diet.

Conclusion: the ketogenic diet undoubtedly has its uses. For those wanting or needing to lose weight fast, it's probably the best diet out there. It's also a proven treatment for people unfortunate enough to have epilepsy.

However, I do have concerns about it. For one, it is a very high-fat diet. If people can restrict that fat intake to the healthier unsaturated fats, all well and good. Unfortunately, many people are going to take this plan as their cue to fill up with more saturated fat than is good for them.

My second concern is that it's just too extreme. Most people simply don't need to lose weight as rapidly as they are likely to with this diet.

Weight Watchers Diet

This diet allows you to eat whatever you want - cheese, cream, biscuits, pasta - nothing is off-limits. However, in order to achieve its goal of making you shed those pounds, it encourages you to plump for more healthy foods.

The basic concept is that all foods are given a rating dependent on their protein, carbohydrate, fat and fibre content. Foods that are good for you have a lower rating than those that are less good. Essentially, the diet steers you toward vegetables, fruit and protein, and away from the fatty, sugary stuff.

Dieters are given a points target that is worked out according to their nutritional profile and what they want to achieve. They can then spend their points on whatever food they like as long as the total spent is within their daily allowance.

An unusual aspect of this diet is the level of support available. Besides the optional meetings and personal coaching, Weight Watchers has an online community, a magazine, and a web site with tools, recipes, tips, success stories and more. There is even a section just for men. You can also sign up online for a newsletter.

Pros: the support network is key for many people as it gives them the encouragement they need to persevere with the diet. The focus on nutritious foods makes it a good choice for people with, or at risk of, high blood pressure, diabetes and heart disease.

Also, the Weight Watchers system encourages daily exercise and rewards it with Fitpoints. These can then be used to buy more, or higher calorie, food. Another advantage is that weight is lost at a slow, steady rate - much healthier than losing half a stone a week or whatever as with some of the more extreme diets.

Cons: Weight Watchers is not free - there is a monthly fee that depends on the level that you choose. If you have a lot of weight to lose, the cost may end up being significant. The need to be always counting points is tedious and time-consuming and soon puts many people off.

Dieters with limited self-control find that being able to eat anything they like is too tempting. Plans that set strict guidelines are better for these people.

Another drawback is that it makes you count points rather than calories. So when coming off the diet, many people quickly put weight back on because they simply don't know the calorific value of food. They may be aware that a plate of fish and chips is worth 14 points but they don't know it contains around 800 calories!

Conclusion: for many people, this diet does work. However, there is a financial cost and, to a large degree, it depends on dieters attending the meetings. For these reasons, it will not be for everyone.

Part Three - Digging Deeper

Nutrition can be a confusing issue with a lot of things to consider. So much so, in fact, that it can be difficult for people who want to improve their diet to know where to start. The blatant misinformation campaigns run by the big food corporations make it even more difficult.

Then there's the Internet - so useful in so many ways but also full of incorrect and outdated information - can you believe what you read?

You should by now have a much clearer idea of the food you're going to have to eat to achieve your goal - be it weight loss or general good health. However, there are still some issues that need clarification and it's these that I'm going to look at in this section of the book.

First up are the labels and ingredient lists on food packaging. The food companies have quite deliberately designed these to be as confusing and unhelpful as possible. I'll show you how to make sense of them.

Superfoods are touted as being very nutritious and thus good for our health. However, not all of them are quite as good as they're cracked up to be. We'll see which these are.

Organic farming is big business and getting more so every day. Supposedly, it produces food that is healthier, not just for us, but also for the environment. It's meant to be much kinder on the animals as well! Are these claims true?

Two relatively new food-preparation techniques are blending (smoothies) and juicing. I'll give you the low-down on both.

Finally, I investigate a dietary strategy known as intermittent fasting and see what it has to offer.

What's In Your Food?

If we all ate the perfect diet, packaged foods simply wouldn't exist - there would be no call for them. However, we don't and they do. There can actually be very few people in the western world who do not eat some form of packaged food. How many of us though, have any idea of what's in that packet, box or tin?

For those of us who don't and would like to, the authorities now compel the food companies to list the ingredients, and also some nutritional information, on the product's packaging. These lists are invariably placed at the rear, or side, of the box. That leaves the front clear for the manufacturer's marketing spiel.

Nutrition Label

On the nutrition label, you will see figures for the amount of calories, fat, sugar, salt, protein and carbohydrates. This is straightforward and so I won't dwell on it. However, I will mention the calorie and sugar counts.

Specified first on the label is the food's calorie count. For millions of overweight people this is probably the most important figure to be aware of. If this includes you, you may be interested to know that the current recommended daily calorie intake is 2,200 - 2,500 calories for men and 1,800 - 2,200 for women.

By using the nutrition labels, you can keep your calorie intake within these limits. This should definitely help in preventing weight gain. The other value everyone should look at is the food's sugar content - quite simply, the lower it is, the better.

Ingredient List

The ingredients in a food are listed in order by their weight. So, in most cases, the first two or three ingredients constitute the bulk of it. The ingredients at the bottom of the list weigh the least and so are negligible.

A good tip is to put foods with a long list of ingredients back on the shelf - inevitably, these will contain many additives that you really shouldn't be eating.

You should be aware the manufacturers try and hide the fact that a food contains sugar by the simple expedient of calling it something else. Names commonly used for this purpose include glucose, fructose, dextrose, sucrose, corn sweetener, sorbitol, high fructose corn syrup, lactose, maltose and sorghum. They may not sound it but these are all sugars!

It's the same with salt. Commonly used names include monosodium glutamate, sodium nitrite, disodium phosphate and sodium benzoate. In fact, any ingredient with 'sodium' in its name is basically salt.

Another trick the food companies use is to try and convince us a product is more nutritious than it actually is. They do this by putting various health claims on the front of the packaging. Two common examples are 'enriched flour' and 'fortified wheat flour'.

Anyone falling for this blurb would assume nutrients of some type have been added to the flour. And they'd be right - the company really has added some vitamins and minerals - typically, iron, calcium, niacin, thiamine, riboflavin and vitamin D.

But what they don't tell you is that these are synthetic minerals and vitamins that have been created in a laboratory. The 'nutrients' are not a patch on the real thing and several studies have shown our bodies struggle to even absorb them, never mind actually use them.

Finally, keep a sharp lookout for the presence of trans fats - these will be listed as either 'hydrogenated oil' or 'partially hydrogenated oil'. Trans fats are bad news as I state repeatedly in the book. While the food manufacturers are gradually phasing out the use of these fats, they are still putting them in foods such as savoury snacks (crackers, biscuits, etc), pies, pizza and margarine. They will be around for a long while yet.

Consumers in the USA should be aware that if a product contains less than one gram of trans fats per serving, the manufacturer does not have to mention it on the ingredient list. While you may think that such a minute amount cannot possibly be dangerous, if it's a food you eat every day, it can add up to a substantial amount over time.

We'll see some more examples of how the food companies use labels to misinform and deceive on pages 155-157.

Superfoods

Superfoods are foods that are considered to be rich in nutrients and so very good for our health. However, there are no set criteria for determining what is and what isn't a superfood. Also, as there is no legal regulation of the term, it can be attributed to practically anything, by anyone. This leaves it open to exploitation.

And exploited it is! One reason for this is the fact that increasing numbers of people are now opting to live a healthy life - a crucial element of which is diet. The food companies are well aware of this trend and, as ever, are keen to cash in.

To this end, many of the claims made for these foods are vastly exaggerated or even deliberately deceptive. While a food may well be healthy in its natural state, the processing it goes through may render it much less so. Green tea is a case in question. When this is sold unadulterated, as it should be, it contains a range of antioxidants. But it is quite common for it to be mixed with inferior teas which make it a much less healthy product. Needless to say, this fact is kept quiet. What may have started out as a superfood is no longer so by the time it hits the shops.

The takeaway therefore, is that you must take all claims regarding the supposed benefits of a superfood with a healthy dose of scepticism. There's a lot of truth in the saying - if it looks to good to be true, it probably is. Also, never underestimate the capacity of big business to hype ordinary products as being something out of this world.

So, with that out of the way, let's take a look at the most popular of these so-called superfoods. Some actually are super and have a place in any eating plan. Others, however, are less so as we'll see.

Eggs

This shouldn't come as a surprise - there are enough nutrients in an egg to turn a single fertilized cell into a baby chicken! Really, what else do you need to know! The protein in eggs is of the highest quality to be found in any food.

Eggs are also a veritable powerhouse of other nutrients. Lutein and zeaxanthin are two good examples - these are carotenoids that lower the risk of age-related macular degeneration. This is one of the main causes of blindness. Another is choline - a nutrient known to enhance brain development and memory.

One egg has approximately 75 calories, 7 grams of protein, 5 grams of fat and 1.5 grams of saturated fat. It also contains iron, vitamins, minerals and the carotenoids. Overall, eggs are the most nutritious food on the planet.

Despite all this, many people are concerned about eating them because of their cholesterol content. This fear dates back many years and was sparked by the high incidence of heart disease associated with the high-fat western diet. However, while eggs do have quite a high amount of cholesterol - 213 mg in a large egg, this isn't, and never has been, a cause of heart disease. As I have noted previously, it is a fact that foods high in cholesterol are very good for your health.

The real culprit is the foods eaten along with eggs - processed meats such as sausage and bacon, bagels, cream cheese and highly sugared coffee, etc. All highly refined stuff loaded with unhealthy chemicals, carbohydrates and trans fats. The egg itself actually has very little to do with it!

Even if it did, the incredible amount of high quality nutrition it provides would far outweigh any negative effects. A related fact here is that eggs contain high levels of omega-3 fats that are known to be heart-protective.

The message to take from this is that eggs are perfectly safe to eat. Their cholesterol content is only an issue for people who already have a high level of it - if this is the case with you, it may be sensible to restrict the number of eggs you eat. Everyone else can eat as many as they like.

Quite apart from the nutrition they provide, eggs are also extremely satiating. For example, a three-egg omelette for breakfast is, by itself, sufficient to keep the average person going until midday. Furthermore, they are relatively low in calories so can definitely be incorporated into any weight loss plan.

You do need to take a bit of care when buying eggs though. They are not all made equal and the major egg producers can be trusted about as far as you can throw them. This is clearly demonstrated by the labels they attach to their eggs - free-range, organic, cage-free and free-roaming are the classic examples. These labels are actually largely meaningless.

Take the free-range label; this can be legally applied to eggs laid by birds that are allowed to forage outside for just a few minutes a day! They are usually fed an unhealthy diet high in grains and synthetic additives but little in the way of nutrients. Furthermore, their living environment is almost always an extremely unpleasant one - over-crowded, dirty and very polluted.

It is a fact that many eggs are contaminated with drugs and chemicals. These are used by the producers to control the diseases caused by the unsanitary conditions the birds are forced to live in. They aren't all bad though. While the eggs from the big producers should be avoided at all costs, there are many smaller outfits that do supply a quality, and ethical, product. These producers allow their birds to forage freely in the wild outdoors and eat their natural diet.

Genuine free-range eggs have darker, orange coloured yolks - this indicates a higher nutrient content. The eggs from the larger outfits, however, almost always have an insipid pale yellow yolk,

The message here is that if you want the best possible return from your egg consumption, you must get the best quality eggs. Don't bother looking in the supermarkets - you won't find them there. Instead, you have to source local egg producers who take the time and trouble to produce the genuine article.

While on the subject of quality, you may be interested in the subject of organic eggs. A genuine organic egg is the ultimate and, ideally, is the only type you should eat. To qualify as organic, it should meet a number of criteria.

The birds should be free-range and fed certified, nutrient-enhanced, organic feed. They are not given drugs such as antibiotics (as they are raised in a healthy environment, they simply don't need them) and they are not exposed to chemicals in the form of pesticides, fungicides and herbicides.

TIP - to determine how fresh an egg is, put it in a pan of water - fresh eggs sink to the bottom, stale eggs don't. If the egg is already cooked, you'll know it's fresh if it's difficult to remove the shell.

When it comes to eating your eggs, ideally they will be eaten raw. This is because many of the nutrients are lost in the cooking process. However, few people are going to eat raw eggs so the next best option is to use the lowest heat you can, which basically means poaching or soft-boiling.

Verdict - eggs are the superfood to beat all superfoods. Quite simply, there is nothing better for you on the entire planet.

Blueberries
This North American fruit has had superfood status for quite a while now. Whether or not it actually is, of one thing there can be no dispute - blueberries are a really excellent source of vitamin K. They are also valued for their high levels of antioxidants, while some advocates claim they protect against cancers, heart disease, and even loss of memory.

With regard to the heart disease claim, a well regarded study in 2012 found that people who ate three or more portions of blueberries a week had a 30 percent lower risk of a heart attack than those who ate them once a month or less.

It is also claimed that blueberries combat high blood pressure and atherosclerosis (the build-up of fatty material inside the arteries). They do this by relaxing the walls of blood vessels and so preventing hardening of the arteries - this is a well known cause of heart attacks and strokes.

A recent study indicated that people given blueberry powder supplements, experience a small but significant drop in blood pressure. However, another recent study done on people with metabolic syndrome (an element of which is high blood pressure) showed no effect on blood pressure at all.

Can blueberries prevent cancer? Well, to date there is very little evidence of this. In laboratory studies on cells and animals, blueberry extracts have been shown to reduce free radical damage that can cause cancer. However, it is not clear how well humans absorb these compounds and whether or not they have a protective effect.

With regard to its beneficial effects on memory, again, there is no conclusive evidence of this. A number of small studies have found a link between blueberry consumption and improved spatial learning and memory. However, most of these relied on small sample groups or animals and so carry no real weight.

Blueberries have a high content of fibre, a fact that makes them important with regard to the issue of digestion. A 2011 study reported that people who ate blueberries every day for six weeks had higher levels of a type of bacteria crucial for the health of the digestive system.

Verdict - Not a superfood. The health claims for blueberries simply cannot be substantiated. That said, there is absolutely no doubt that they are extremely good for us, as they are low in calories and high in important nutrients. But then, so are most fruits!

Broccoli

A somewhat unappetising mainstay of school dinners for a long time, broccoli has undergone a resurgence recently. The vegetable is a very good source of fibre, vitamins, omega-3 fatty acids, protein, zinc, calcium, iron, niacin and selenium, to name just some.

Supposedly, it helps fight diseases such as high blood pressure, diabetes, heart disease and cancer. What's the reality though?

With regard to diabetes, broccoli has a high content of an antioxidant called sulforaphane. This may help to alleviate the damage to small blood vessels caused by high blood sugar, as is commonly seen in people with diabetes. There is no conclusive proof of this, though. Another claim made for sulforaphane is that it can inhibit the development of colon and prostate cancers. Again, though, there is no conclusive proof of this.

There is no evidence to support claims that broccoli lowers blood pressure either. A 2010 study in which blood pressure patients were given broccoli for four weeks, found it made no difference whatsoever.

Verdict - Not a superfood. However, it does provide a range of nutrients needed for many of the body's functions. It *may* also offer a small degree of protection against cancer and cardiovascular disease due to its sulforaphane content.

Oily Fish

Oily fish are a very good source of vitamin D, protein, B vitamins and selenium. They are also high in omega-3 fatty acids. This is a type of fat that's very good for our health and which most people don't get nearly enough of.

It's a known fact that Eskimos have a much lower incidence of cardiovascular disease than we do. It's also a fact that they have a diet high in oily fish. So not surprisingly this has sparked research into the health benefits offered by oily fish. The results show quite clearly that fish like salmon, mackerel, tuna and sardines do offer protection against this disease.

Furthermore, they also lower blood pressure. The evidence is conclusive enough for the UK government to recommend that people should eat at least two portions of fish a week, one of which should be an oily type.

There is also evidence to show that eating oily fish several times a week reduces the risk of age-related macular degeneration - a common cause of blindness in older people. However, a study to see whether fish oil supplements could reduce the progression of macular degeneration in people who already had the condition failed to find any evidence that it did.

A study in 2012 looked to see if omega-3 fats could reduce the risk of dementia. The conclusion was that there is no preventative effect.

With regard to prostate cancer, there is some evidence to suggest eating oily fish may reduce the chances of developing it. However, there have been other studies that found no evidence of this.

Verdict - Definitely a superfood. Eating oily fish offers clear and proven protection against cardiovascular disease. It's good for you in many other ways as well. The only reservation is that our oceans are polluted with toxins such as mercury. For this reason, we recommend you eat small varieties such as sardines (tinned or fresh) which don't live long enough to be affected by the toxins. Two or three servings a week is all you need.

Green Tea
After water, tea is the most popular beverage in the world. In the western nations, green tea accounts for about fifteen percent of all tea consumed. Interestingly, few people are aware that, regardless of the various names given to them, all teas come from the same plant - an evergreen shrub called Camellia Sinensis.

What differentiates the various types of tea is the method of production - to be specific, the degree of oxidation they are exposed to. Black teas are exposed to a high level of oxidation whereas green teas are not. The lower level of oxidation is thought to result in less of the tea's nutrients being lost during the manufacturing process.

Green tea is an excellent source of a powerful family of antioxidants called polyphenols, a range of vitamins, and minerals such as zinc and selenium. Popular in Chinese medicine for centuries, it has been used to treat a whole range of ailments.

Elevated fairly recently to the list of so-called superfoods, just what is green tea really good for though? Well, if you believe everything you read, quite a lot actually. It offers protection against cancer and Alzheimer's disease, aids in weight loss, and lowers blood pressure which, if true, means it will help people suffering from cardiovascular disease.

Lets look at the cancer claim first. Eight years ago, a major review of data taken from some fifty separate studies and involving 1.5 million participants, tried to find a link between green tea and cancers of the bowel, prostate, mouth and lungs. None was found.

With regard to Alzheimer's disease, green tea is claimed to be an effective method of treatment due to its high level of antioxidants. However, there is no conclusive evidence to back this up.

Green tea contains a powerful antioxidant called catechin, which is said to promote weight loss by increasing the body's metabolism. This causes calories to be burnt at a faster rate. One study has claimed people who drink green tea burn up to an extra 70-100 calories per day. It neglected to say how much green tea they had to consume to achieve this though!

Most blood pressure drugs work by reducing the effects of a enzyme called Angiotension II. Compounds in green tea are touted as having the same capability. A 2014 survey of data taken from previous studies found evidence of a modest reduction in blood pressure in people who consumed green tea. It was not enough to be considered significant though.

Verdict - Not a superfood. It's a pleasant drink and very good for us in a number of ways. But that's it.

Kale

Kale has rapidly established itself as one of the most popular health foods. A member of the cruciferous vegetable family, it comes with a lot of nutrients. These include vitamins (A, C and K in particular), fibre, protein (unusual in a vegetable) and omega-3 fats.

The health benefits claimed for kale is too long to list here but the main ones are that it has excellent anti-inflammatory properties, it fights a number of cancers, is effective against diabetes, can improve eyesight and is good for heart health.

The reason touted for it being so effective as an anti-inflammatory agent is that it is high in vitamin K. While there is no dispute about this, the fact is all other dark green leafy vegetables are high in vitamin K as well. There is absolutely nothing special about kale in this respect.

With regard to cancer, studies show that compounds found in kale can help fight a range of them, including breast, lung, bladder, colon and liver. However, these have all been done on rodents. Studies done on humans show mixed results - some showing a link and others not showing any.

Kale is good source of antioxidants. These fight free radicals in the body that are considered to cause diseases such as diabetes. They do work. However, once again, *all* fruits and vegetables are high in antioxidants, and so have the same beneficial effect with regard to diabetes and other diseases. This applies to heart disease as well.

Good eyesight is another trumpeted benefit of kale. This is because it is high in carotenoids such as lutein and zeaxanthin. These promote vision and the health of the retina. But, once again, it turns out that while this is true, it is also true of all dark green leafy vegetables.

Verdict - Kale is definitely not a superfood. Like all cruciferous vegetables, it is very good for you but that's as far as it goes - there is absolutely nothing stand-out about it.

Nuts

Packed with protein, minerals, vitamins and fibre; nuts, just like eggs, are powerhouses of nutrition. There are many types, most offering both general, and specific, health benefits. One thing common to all of them is a very high fat content. It's the fear that this will make them put on weight that prevents many people from eating nuts.

However, studies have shown quite clearly that eating nuts does not cause weight gain - in fact, as part of a sensible and controlled diet, they will actually do the opposite - make you lose weight. This is because they are satiating and so stop you feeling hungry.

As nuts are such an important source of high quality nutrients, I'll take a brief look at the main types and see what they have to offer:

Almonds - almonds are a great source of bone-building calcium and so are ideal for people who don't eat dairy products for whatever reason. They are also high in vitamin E and other antioxidants that nourish the skin and reduce signs of aging.

Almonds have compounds called flavonoids in their skin that are known to improve artery health and reduce inflammation - good for maintaining a healthy heart. Almonds are also the best source of protein of all the nuts.

Brazil Nuts - a key nutrient provided by brazil nuts

is a mineral called selenium. This is critical to several body functions that include prevention of damage to the thyroid gland, combating inflammation, and DNA production. It's also important for the liver and kidneys.

Three nuts a day provides all the selenium you need. Brazil nuts are high in calories and so are a good source of instant energy - this makes them ideal for people who are active.

Cashews - Cashews are a very rich source of minerals - copper and magnesium especially. The latter is known to be important for brain function, memory recall, reducing the risk of migraine attacks and keeping blood pressure under control.

Copper is used in the production of skin, bone and hair pigments called melanin and collagen. Amongst many other things, these help provide our skin's elasticity.

Cashews also contain flavanols that inhibit the ability of cancer cells to divide and multiply, so reducing the incidence of some types of cancer.

Chestnuts - nutrition-wise, there's nothing that special about chestnuts. They do, however, have an extremely high level of fibre which makes them a low-glycemic index food. Accordingly, they can help manage glucose levels in people with type 2 diabetes.

They also have less fat and calories than any other nut. This makes them an ideal addition to a weight-loss diet. When ground up, they form a gluten-free flour that can be used for baking.

Hazelnuts - hazelnuts are rich in potassium, calcium and magnesium - minerals that provide a number of health benefits. A very important one of these is the maintenance of healthy blood pressure.

Hazelnuts are also rich in oleic acid - this is known to lower blood sugar and insulin levels and helps minimise the effects of diabetes.

Pecans - just one ounce of pecans provides 10 percent of the recommended daily amount of fibre. They are also one of the most antioxidant-rich foods in the world.

As with hazelnuts, pecans are high in oleic acid and so are good for diabetes sufferers. Many of the minerals found in pecans contribute to the proper functioning of the brain.

Recent research has found that some nutrients in pecans can be helpful to people suffering from osteoporosis. They do this by increasing bone mass and reducing bone loss.

Walnuts - of all the nuts, walnuts are the best with

regard to heart health. This is because of their rich content of omega-3, 6 and 9 fats. Omega-3 is also known to be good for cognitive function, which means walnuts feed the brain as well

Studies have shown that a handful of walnuts a day cuts the risk of both prostate and breast cancer. The same handful also has a significant impact on male fertility, i.e. sperm quality. This is one of the lesser known benefits of walnuts.

Pistachios - native to the Middle East, pistachios are lower in calories than most nuts - this makes them ideal for people who are trying to lose weight as well as improve their diet. Nutrition-wise, as with nuts in general, they provide a range of minerals plus a large amount of protein.

However, one issue with these nuts is that the majority of them are bleached before being put on sale. This is done to hide unsightly staining on the shells caused by the harvesting process. Not only can this leave bleach residues on the nuts, important phytochemicals in their skins are destroyed. For this reason, I recommend you eat only organically grown pistachio nuts.

Macadamias - macadamias are the most nutrient-rich of all the nuts. They are also low in carbohydrates and protein while being high in omega-3 fatty acids.

100 grams of macadamias provides 25 percent of the daily recommended amount of fibre. They are also a very good source of phytosterols that help regulate cholesterol levels. They are, however, the nut with the highest calorie count.

Verdict - Superfood. Nuts are a superb source of unsaturated fats, vitamin E, antioxidants, omega-3 fatty acids and fibre. This makes them one of the most nutritious foods on the planet. Eating a handful of mixed nuts every day is one of the best things you can do if you are seeking a long and healthy life.

Avocados

Native to Central and South America and classified as a fruit, avocados are yet another of nature's products that positively brim with health-giving nutrients.

As with nuts, these green fruits are an excellent source of monounsaturated fats. They provide close to twenty essential nutrients, including potassium, vitamins A, C and E, folic acid and B-vitamins. They are a rich source of potassium (twice the amount found in bananas) and folic acid. The fruits also provide a high amount of fibre, which is another very good reason to eat them.

Benefits claimed for avocados include weight control, protection against cancer, heart disease and anti-inflammatory properties.

How good are they though? Well, firstly, the high content of monounsaturated fats makes avocados extremely satiating so you don't feel the need to eat so much (one avocado provides half of your daily fibre requirement). Not only that, they provide a lot of energy - this enables you to cut down on carbohydrates should your weight be an issue.

The high fat content also enables you to more efficiently absorb fat-soluble nutrients from other foods eaten in conjunction. Furthermore, it is a well-known fact that monounsaturated fat offers protection against heart disease and also lowers blood pressure.

With regard to cancer, several studies have been done in an attempt to find a link. One of these concluded that phytochemicals in avocados make them *potentially* beneficial for inhibiting the development of prostate and oral cancer. A 2014 Chinese study showed an antioxidant called lutein, which is high in avocados, may reduce the risk of developing breast cancer.

While there is nothing conclusive at the time of writing, there is considerable excitement at the potential benefits offered by avocados in the prevention and treatment of cancer.

Avocados contain chemicals called phytosterols that have anti-inflammatory properties known to be good for treating osteoarthritis - this is a condition suffered by some eight million people in the UK alone.

Verdict - Superfood. Avocados contain too many healthy fats and nutrients, such as oleic acid, lutein, folate, vitamins, monounsaturated fats, fibre and antioxidants, to be anything but.

Tip - many of the nutrients found in avocados are in the dark green part of the fruit just under the skin.

Chia Seeds

Originating in Mexico, chia seeds are becoming one of the most popular foods with the health-conscious. This is hardly surprising when you consider the huge array of nutrients they offer. These include protein, vitamins, antioxidants, fibre, healthy fats and minerals.

So what are they good for? Well, if you believe the claims made for them, they have anti-aging properties, are good for the heart, the digestive system, bones and teeth, plus they help with diabetes and weight loss.

Chia seeds have a high content of antioxidants which neutralise free radicals (damaged body cells) that, amongst other things, cause damage to the skin and aging in general. So they may be helpful in these respects. There is no proof of this though.

Chia seeds provide more omega-3 fats than salmon. This has led many people to think they must, therefore, be very good for the heart. However, while they undoubtedly are, it's a fact that plant-based omega-3 fats are not as good as those from animal sources.

With a high fibre content, chia seeds can be nothing else than extremely good for our digestive systems. There is no dispute here.

With regard to bones and teeth, they do have a high level of the necessary nutrients - protein, calcium, magnesium and phosphorus. In fact, chia seeds provide more calcium than most dairy products. This makes them a very good source of this essential mineral for people who don't eat dairy for whatever reason.

There is research that suggests chia seeds lower blood sugar levels and so can help control diabetes. However, there is no evidence that this is actually the case.

Verdict - Chia seeds *may* be a superfood. The main issue with the many health claims made for them is the lack of conclusive evidence. The few studies done have been mainly on animals. However, superfood or not, they do make a very worthwhile addition to any diet.

Coconut Oil

The coconut tree is thought to originate in South America. The oil, taken from the pressed meat of the coconuts, has only recently gained superfood status. Bear this fact in mind when you evaluate the various claims made for its supposed benefits. These include weight loss, heart health, treating Alzheimer's, improving digestion and many others.

Coconut oil contains more saturated fat than butter, beef tallow and lard (no less than ninety percent of it is fat). It has no carbohydrates or protein and only minute amounts of a few assorted nutrients.

However, as I've mentioned elsewhere, saturated fat is not the demon it's made out to be - it is, in fact, very good for us - *in small amounts*. So when consumed in said small amounts, the fat content of coconut oil is nothing to be alarmed about. That's the first thing.

The second is that 50 percent of this saturated fat is lauric acid - a medium-chain fatty acid (MCFA) that has several health-promoting properties. One of these is that it increases the rate we burn calories. For this reason, coconut oil is being touted as a means of losing weight and a recent study has suggested that this might actually be the case. However, it only involved a few subjects so cannot be taken too seriously.

Still with lauric acid, when the liver breaks it down, ketones are created that can be used as fuel by the brain. There is a current theory that because these ketones supply energy to the brain thus eliminating the need for insulin to convert glucose into energy, coconut oil is an effective treatment for people with Alzheimer's. While there may be something in this, a study has yet to be done that actually proves it.

MCFAs are also thought to boost digestive health. This is because they are easily absorbed in the digestive tract, plus they apparently help other nutrients to be absorbed as well. If so, it follows that people with digestive disorders like Crohn's disease will benefit from eating coconut oil.

Verdict - Not a superfood by any stretch of the imagination. There are no conclusive studies that prove otherwise. In fact, for some people coconut oil could even be dangerous due to its extremely high content of saturated fat. If you're looking for a healthy oil, go with olive oil which has proven benefits.

Turmeric
A spice native to Southern Asia, turmeric has a deep orange-gold colour and is widely used for cooking and as a colouring agent (it is the main ingredient in curry powder). Before use, it is usually dried, boiled and then

ground into a powder.

It has been used for centuries in China where it is thought to have medicinal qualities.

One of the main claims made for turmeric is that it is rich in a compound called curcumin - this is thought to give it anti-inflammatory properties. Indeed, there are studies that indicate curcumin may be effective at fighting Alzheimer's disease and cancer.

Other studies show it has a high content of antioxidants that fight and neutralise the free radicals in our bodies that can be the cause of so many illnesses.

However, it's a known fact that turmeric is not easily absorbed by the body. Therefore, to get any worthwhile benefits from it, assuming there are any, you would need to consume so much of the stuff there would almost certainly be side effects. It is also a fact that many of the studies done have involved conflicts of interest, i.e. researchers with vested interests in the results.

Verdict - Not a superfood. As is so often the case, the claims made for this undoubtedly tasty spice are overblown. There simply aren't any studies that provide conclusive proof for any of them.

The Best Foods To Eat

Having established which of the superfoods actually are super, I'll now take a look at foods the health benefits of which are beyond doubt. If everybody ate these foods and nothing else, the human race would be infinitely healthier.

Meat

Red meat first. Much vilified these days due to its saturated fat content that supposedly causes high blood pressure, heart disease and obesity, red meat is actually one of the most nutrient-rich foods on the planet.

This is why nature designed the human body to eat it - we are, in fact, genetically programmed to function at the optimal level on a diet that includes red meat. Most animals, and many birds, eat it as well and for the same reason.

Red meat provides us with high-quality protein that contains all the amino acids required for building muscle and bone. It is also an excellent source of B vitamins - these are essential for our brains. Lack of them can cause confusion, impaired senses, aggression, insomnia, weakness, dementia and peripheral neuropathy.

In addition, it is rich in zinc which supports the immune system, and iron which builds red blood cells and gives us energy.

You may have seen meat labelled as 'organic', 'free range' and 'grass fed' and be wondering if it is worth paying extra for. This is a relatively new and expanding market fuelled by people's understandable desire to eat more healthily.

Unfortunately, like virtually all food markets, it is riddled with false and unsubstantiated claims. Yes, these animals may have more space than their factory-farmed cousins, but mostly they're subjected to the same unhappy regime of high-energy feed, selective breeding for rapid weight gain and minimal exercise.

The truth is, nutrition-wise, these meats are only slightly better for you than factory-farmed meat and, all other things being equal, are most definitely not worth the premium you will pay for them.

That said, should you be lucky enough to find the genuine article (and you will be lucky!) you will at least get meat that is free of the steroids, antibiotics and growth hormones found in factory-farmed meat.

With regard to white meat (chicken, turkey, duck, etc) the only real difference between it and red meat is the colour and flavour. Nutrition-wise, there's little between them. They are both extremely good for us when eaten in sensible quantities.

Seafood

With a similar level of proteins and minerals, meat that comes from the sea has much the same nutritional value as red and white meat. However, in comparison, it offers only small to moderate amounts of vitamins.

Where seafood does have an advantage is its fat content - lower than in red meat. Furthermore, one of these fats is the healthy polyunsaturated omega-3 fat. As I have already mentioned, this is thought to play an important role in lowering the risk of heart disease.

Fatty fish, such as herring, mackerel, sardines, salmon and tuna, all provide a good amount of omega-3 fat and are, indeed, one of the best sources of it.

Being low in fat means seafood is also low in calories, so eating it is much better than eating meat if you are looking to lose weight.

However, there are a couple of caveats with regard to eating fish. The first is that we have contaminated the oceans with pollutants such as mercury and dioxin. As a result, many fish now have dangerous amounts of this toxic stuff and so should be avoided completely. These are the larger fish, such as albacore tuna, swordfish, king mackerel and sharks.

Smaller sea creatures lower down on the food chain are much safer as they don't live long enough to absorb dangerous amounts of these pollutants. These include sardines, anchovies, crab, shrimps, prawns and oysters, etc.

The second caveat is the issue of fish farming. There is actually a world of difference between farm-raised fish and those caught in the wild. Farmed fish are raised in filthy, over-crowded conditions that cause diseases and parasites. To control these diseases, they are given antibiotics, and for the parasites they are given pesticides.

These unfortunate creatures are fed a totally unnatural diet that consists mainly of grain-based pellets. This gives them nutrition levels that are much lower than those of wild-caught fish. For example, farmed salmon may be much fattier than wild salmon, but they contain much less healthy omega-3 fats and protein.

Be aware that industrial fish farming is the fastest growing form of food production in the world. Approximately 50 percent (and rising) of the world's seafood now comes from it. Don't let this put you off fish though - I urge you to eat it. Just be sure to eat the right types and get them from the right sources.

Dairy Produce
Diary products are basically butter, cheese, milk, yoghurt and cream. We'll start with the most commonly consumed type - milk.

Of the three versions of milk commonly found in the shops - full-fat (whole), semi-skimmed and skimmed - the only one worth consuming is full-fat. Skimmed milk has all the cream (fat) removed and semi-skimmed milk has a lesser amount removed.

The removal of the fat renders skimmed milk almost totally devoid of nutritional value. This is because the vitamins in milk are fat-soluble, meaning they need fat in order to be absorbed by the body. Without the fat it is, essentially, little more than water.

Furthermore, the fat also gives milk its flavour and texture - removing it makes it bland and tasteless. It's also a fact that because skimmed milk is a highly processed food, it will usually leave you feeling unsatisfied and wanting something more.

Full-fat milk, however, is totally different. As a result of being stigmatised for years by various government advisory bodies (most of which are in the pocket of the processed food industry), many people have been put off drinking it due to the supposed dangers of its saturated fat content.

However, it is precisely because of that fat content (including the fat-soluble vitamins A, D, E and K) that it is in fact extremely good for you. Amongst other things, full-fat milk strengthens immunity to infections and provides calcium that helps keep bones healthy.

It's also a fact that full-fat milk is not actually a high-fat food. As a general rule, anything with a fat content of 20 percent or over is considered to be high-fat, but full-fat milk only contains between 3 percent and 5 percent.

Less commonly available is organic and raw milk. Organic milk is produced without the use of pesticides and with higher standards of animal welfare than non-organic. Accordingly, it is more nutritious as the cows eat what nature intended them to eat - green grass. It offers higher levels of omega-3 fats, vitamin E, iron and other nutrients.

Raw milk is the real deal - unadulterated and straight from the cow, just as nature intended it to be. As with organic, it comes from grass-fed cows and is unpasteurized and unhomogenized. As a result, raw milk retains all of its natural enzymes, fatty acids, vitamins and minerals. This makes it one of the most nutrient-dense foods in the world. It also tastes wonderful and has a rich, creamy consistency.

It has, however, attracted a lot of bad publicity because it is unpasteurized and so is supposedly unsafe to drink. The fact that this publicity is largely driven by the processed food industry, which sees no advantage, i.e. profit, in raw milk should give the lie to this though.

As should the fact that man has been drinking raw milk for thousands of years without any problems at all.

As long as it is purchased from a reputable source, raw milk is perfectly safe and far more nutritious than any other type.

So, drink as much raw, organic and full-fat milk as you like and give the skimmed versions a definite miss - they are little more than water and will do you no good at all.

Moving on to cheese, as with milk, this food has been vilified for years due to its high fat content. Again though, as with milk, it is actually extremely good for you and provides a whole host of vitamins (particularly K2), plus minerals and protein.

It should go without saying by now that the most nutritious and flavoursome cheeses are the ones made from the milk of grass-fed animals. Sadly, the vast majority of cheeses sold in the stores aren't and so are inferior. That said, they are still well worth eating - just not as good.

Do not, however, be tempted by the many types of processed cheese on the market. By this, I mean products such as individually wrapped cheeses, spreadable cheese, sliced cheese, string cheese and spray cheese. These should be given a very wide berth. Not only are they bland and tasteless, they are actually very bad for you.

Check out the ingredients on the box of one of these cheeses and you will see a long list that includes stuff like dairy by-products, emulsifiers, sodium, saturated vegetable oils, preservatives, colouring agents and sugar, to name just some.

Real cheese is a simple fermented dairy product made from just a few ingredients and which can be identified by its label. Examples are blue cheese, cheddar cheese, camembert and brie. As with all real cheeses, these need to be kept in a refrigerator.

Also subject to the 'fat is bad' school of thought is butter. Along with milk and cheese, this has received a bad press over the years. However, it is actually an excellent source of vitamins such as A, D and K, which play an important role in the efficient absorption of calcium.

These vitamins are also beneficial to the body's immune system, and are thought to play a role in the suppression of cancer cell growth. Also found in butter is a compound called sodium butyrate. Recent studies show this is effective in the treatment and prevention of diet-induced insulin resistance.

However, none of these benefits are provided by the products that masquerade as butter. Here, I am talking about margarine, shortening and the 'spreads' of various kinds. These all contain trans fats which, as I have stated repeatedly, are extremely dangerous and should not be eaten.

Eggs

There are two points to be made with regard to eggs. The first is the high level of cholesterol in the yolks, and the second is the unbelievable amount of nutrients they provide.

The first issue, cholesterol, has been covered on pages 39-43 so I won't go into it again here.

Moving on to their nutritional content, eggs are a very good source of high quality protein. More than half of this is found in the whites, along with vitamin B2, and low amounts of fat and cholesterol. The whites are also rich sources of selenium, vitamins D, B6, B12 and minerals such as zinc, iron and copper.

The yolks have a higher content of calories and fat and, apart from being an egg's main source of cholesterol, are also its main source of the fat soluble vitamins A, D, E and K, and lecithin.

Eggs also contain lutein and zeaxanthin. As we have already seen, these antioxidants have major benefits for eye health and significantly reduce the risk of cataracts and macular degeneration - both very common eye disorders.

Yet another benefit of eating eggs is the fact they're

extremely satiating - this makes them the ideal food to include in a weight-loss diet.

The bottom line then is that eggs are the most nutritious food on planet Earth - nothing else comes even close. Eat them to your heart's content.

Vegetables
Most vegetables are very low in calories and carbs while, at the same time, having a high content of the fibre, vitamins and minerals your body needs to achieve and maintain optimal health.

Vegetables reduce the risk of getting a range of chronic diseases, such as heart disease, stroke, diabetes and even some cancers. Not only that, they are good for improving cognitive function and are effective against Alzheimer's disease, kidney stones and digestive issues. Furthermore, they provide antioxidants and compounds that aren't found in any other type of food.

Some vegetables are better for you than others. These are the cruciferous vegetables such as cabbage and green leafy vegetables like kale. Not only are they very high in fibre, they also have the lowest content of carbohydrates - this makes them the ideal food for a weight-loss diet. Other vegetables in this category include beet greens, brussels sprouts, cauliflowers, bell peppers, broccoli, eggplant and spinach.

Root vegetables are of lesser value as, typically, they have less fibre. Also, being more starchy, they have higher levels of carbs. So, while still very good for you, their leafy cousins have the edge thanks to their higher fibre content.

And, of course, if weight is a factor then the carb content of root vegetables becomes an issue, particularly with potatoes. Once again, the leafy vegetables will be the ones to go for.

In both categories of vegetable, there is a huge range to choose from. So which are the best ones to eat?

Of the leafy vegetables, the general consensus is that kale offers most benefits, closely followed by spinach, mustard greens, swiss chard, arugula and romaine lettuce.

With regard to root vegetables, it's butternut squash, sweet potatoes, carrots, parsnips, beets, ginger, turmeric and eggplant.

Fruit

From a nutritional viewpoint, fruit in general offers much the same in the way of nutrients as vegetables do. They have similar levels of vitamins, minerals, fibre and health-enhancing compounds such as antioxidants.

The drawback with fruit is the fact that it has a high sugar content - a type of sugar known as fructose. As we have already established, eating too much sugar leads to excess weight which, in turn, is the cause of a large number of illnesses and chronic diseases.

Now when eaten in small quantities, there is nothing wrong with fructose. But because it is routinely added to commonly taken sweeteners such as honey and table sugar, and virtually all processed foods, most people are eating far more of it than is good for them.

This is just one part of the problem - another is that the body handles fructose differently than it does other sugars. For example, eating glucose triggers an increase in the production of insulin, which enables the glucose to be used for energy. Glucose consumption also increases production of leptin, which regulates appetite and fat storage in the body.

Neither of these processes happen when you eat fructose, so the net effect is that it gets stored as fat.

People in good health, who aren't overweight and aren't insulin resistant, can eat fruit without problem. Indeed, it is recommended that they do. However, people who are overweight, have diabetes, high blood pressure or a high level of cholesterol are advised to limit the amount of fruit they eat. Either that or drastically reduce the amount of processed food they eat!

With regard to which fruits are best to eat, you won't

go wrong with berries, avocados, olives, papayas, mangoes, pineapples, bananas and kiwifruit.

Berries are probably the best fruit of all as they offer all the nutrients and fibre that other fruits do but without the high level of sugar. Of the berries, blueberries, raspberries and blackberries are probably the pick of the bunch.

Also well worth a mention are avocados. These tropical fruits are an excellent source of healthy fats, fibre, potassium, folate, and a wide range of vitamins. Indeed, as I point out on pages 88-90, avocados are considered to be a superfood.

Those of you looking for fruits low in carbs need look no further than berries (not blueberries, though), watermelon, cantaloupes and coconuts.

Now we come to the fruits to avoid. Lets start with the seedless varieties. These are fruits that have been artificially developed so that they have no seeds. As consumption of these fruits is generally easier and more convenient, this is considered to give them added commercial value. Various methods are used to create them, such as genetic modification and grafting.

While, currently, there is no evidence that they are in any way bad for us, they simply haven't been around long enough for the long-term effects of regular consumption to be evaluated. For this reason, I suggest you don't eat them.

It's also worth pointing out that much of a plant's nutritional content, be it a fruit or a vegetable, is concentrated in its seeds. So while a seedless fruit may be more convenient to eat, it will not be nearly as nutritious as nature intended it to be.

Then we have dried fruit. This is fruit that has had its water content removed so creating an extremely high sugar content. As long as it is eaten in small quantities though, it won't be a problem. Just remember that being a processed food, dried fruit usually has preservatives, sugar, vegetable oils and goodness knows what else added to it.

Legumes

A legume is a dry fruit that grows inside a seed or pod. The most well-known of these are peas, beans and lentils. They are all excellent sources of healthy fats, protein, fibre and carbs - albeit in small amounts.

The most common type of legume is the beans. These include broad beans, black beans, mung beans, soybeans, navy beans, chickpeas, kidney beans and lima beans. They are all high in carbs and protein but low in fat.

Some legumes are called peas. These include green peas, snow peas, snap peas, split peas and black-eyed peas.

Similar to beans, peas contain high concentrations of carbohydrates, fibre and protein, but little fat.

Lentils are round, oval or heart-shaped seeds, usually split into halves. They are available in a number of varieties that differ in colour, texture and taste. The most common of these are the black, green, and red varieties. Black lentils, also known as beluga, are famous for their similarity to caviar.

The two things that all types of legume have in common are their high levels of protein and fibre. For people who don't eat meat, or restrict their intake of it, this high protein content makes them an ideal substitute for the protein they're not getting from the meat.

As for the fibre content, this is great for those on a diet. A spoonful every now and then keeps those hunger pangs at bay, thus restricting the urge to eat.

Note that some legumes are incorrectly called nuts. The most common example of this is the peanut - others being soy nuts and carob nuts.

Summary
The foods I have just talked about - meat, eggs, seafood, dairy produce, nuts, vegetables, fruit and legumes, contain *all* the nutrients required for optimum health. You need eat nothing else!

The same cannot be said for the foods I look at in the next section. Eat these on a regular basis, as so many people do, and you'll be heading for an early grave - it's your choice!

Foods & Drinks to Avoid

The processed food industry is now reckoned to be just about the largest industry on Earth and is estimated to generate some two trillion pounds per annum. This has not happened by accident - the food companies have achieved it by deception, dishonesty, clever marketing and swiftly latching onto, and exploiting, the various food trends and fads as they emerge.

The latest of these is health food. However, this has presented them with a problem - processed food is inherently unhealthy, and always will be. So in order to cash in, they have had to resort, once again, to deception.

Two methods have been used. The first has been the creation of foods aimed specifically at the health-conscious, such as energy bars and drinks. The second is to take existing foods that are known to be unhealthy and, seemingly, make them healthy.

What they don't tell you though, is that while the energy bars and drinks do provide a boost of energy, they also provide an unhealthy dose of sugar and often an almost total lack of nutrients.

When they claim to have made an unhealthy food healthy, they've done it by taking out the saturated fat.

This enables them to say the food is now low in calories and so healthy. What they don't say, however, is that they've replaced the fat with a cocktail of chemicals designed to replicate the taste and texture provided by the fat. The end result is something that appears to be a health food but is actually riddled with chemicals and so is anything but.

Then there's all the other foods that people know are not good for them but, because they love them so much, they keep on eating. There's simply no incentive for the manufacturers to improve them - if the people are happy to eat rubbish, they're happy to sell it to them!

So, lets see some classic examples of the food companies dishonesty and indifference:

Energy Bars
The advertising blurb on the packaging of these products invariably extols how low in calories they are and the huge amount of protein and fibre they provide. This makes them seem like a super-healthy option - an impression reinforced by the fact they're sold in health food shops and many gyms.

Some of them do actually live up to the hype by being low in saturated fat and sugars, and offering a decent amount of protein and fibre. This makes them a nutritious and satisfying pick-me-up. Unfortunately, these bars are the exception - most are actually the exact opposite.

This is because they consist largely of artificial sweeteners and cereals all wrapped in an outer layer designed to look healthy and appetising. While they do provide a quick energy boost, in the long-term, use of these bars will cause the pounds to pile on.

One of the sweeteners used are sugar alcohols, due to them being low in calories. However, they are difficult for our bodies to digest and can cause wind, bloating and diarrhoea.

The so-called protein content is often a blatant con. Cheap soy and whey proteins are usually used; the low qualities of which are, in any case, largely destroyed by the production process.

Synthetic vitamins go in the mix as well. These are cheap and allow labelling such as 'fortified with' to be used.

The bottom line is that there's actually little point to energy bars. They're not much different to the average candy bar which also provides an energy boost. They are a lot more expensive though!

Energy & Sports Drinks
Possibly even worse than energy bars are the energy

& sports drinks. Typically, these include caffeine, sugar, amino acids, synthetic vitamins, herbal supplements and taurine. According to the advertising, they provide a boost to stamina, endurance and mental concentration.

While they no doubt do, to some degree at any rate, they also have less desirable effects. For one, their phenomenally high content of sugar is a known cause of obesity - this can lead to type 2 diabetes. Others are high blood pressure, convulsions, nausea and vomiting. These drinks are also very rich in caffeine.

Some contain as much as 20 teaspoons of sugar, believe it or not! This is three times the recommended daily maximum for an adult. While sugar-free versions are available, they are still loaded with caffeine with some having four times as much as a cup of coffee.

As caffeine is a powerful stimulant, overuse can cause a number of problems that include heart palpitations, insomnia, hallucinations, anxiety and stomach ulcers.

As if all this wasn't bad enough, the high sugar and caffeine content means energy drinks are also addictive.

Soft Drinks
Along with the energy drinks, soft fizzy drinks are just about the worst thing you can put into your body. They may look and taste good but they have virtually no

nutritional value.

To start with, they increase the risk of getting cancer - pancreatic cancer in particular. This is due to the high sugar content which forces the pancreas to increase its production of insulin.

Fizzy soft drinks can cause hyperactivity by altering the protein levels in the brain. This is thought to be caused by the flavourings and colourings used in the drinks.

They contain a large amount of caffeine. This causes the same health issues that the energy drinks do, although perhaps to a lesser degree.

Another major ingredient is phosphoric acid. This can restrict the body's ability to absorb and use calcium, which leads to osteoporosis (softening of the teeth and bones). Note that caffeine is also known to interfere with calcium absorption and so may contribute to this issue as well.

Packed with sugar, soft drinks are one of the major causes of the current obesity crisis. Obesity, is of course, the trigger for a range of illnesses and diseases. And don't assume the so-called 'diet' versions are any better - they aren't. This is because they are sweetened with artificial sweeteners, a typical example being aspartame - 200 times sweeter than sugar!

The problem with these artificial sweeteners is that no one has a clue with regard to their long term effects. In any case, all the evidence so far indicates that diet drinks actually cause weight gain. While no one knows why precisely, it is thought to have something to do with the way the our brains react to the artificial sweeteners.

To sum up, carbonated soft drinks are a known cause of dangerous conditions that include heart disease, cancer, osteoporosis, obesity and non-alcoholic fatty liver disease. Oh, and they rot your teeth as well! Give your body a break - drink something else.

Ice Cream

This one will surprise a lot of people. Ice cream is one of the most popular snacks in the world and has been for many many years. However, that's because very few people know what goes into it these days. Years ago, ice cream was a healthy enough blend of little more than frozen double cream, milk, sugar, lard and eggs.

Then the big food companies got in on the act. Now, it bears little resemblance to the ice cream of old. If you read the label on a tub, you'll see a long list of ingredients that reads something like: milk, sugar, corn syrup, whey, mono and diglycerides, carob bean gum, guar gum, carrageenan, natural flavour, annatto (for colour), vitamin A palmitate and tara gum. Not quite the same is it!

Many ice creams now don't even contain cream and, in some cases, no milk either. Instead, the producers use vegetable oil - typically, palm oil which is high in saturated fat and one of the unhealthiest vegetable oils on the planet!

In the UK, the amount of dairy produce the manufacturers must put in ice cream in order to be able to legally call it such, is extremely low - a minimum of 2.5 percent milk and 5 percent dairy fat. And if you think that's bad, it gets worse!

Rather than use good quality protein, they use whey solids - a low-grade protein which is a waste product of the cheese industry. In fact, for a long time this was just dumped into the rivers and seas - it had zero commercial value.

Also, ice cream is sold by volume, not weight. So it's bulked it out by whipping as much air into the mixture as possible before freezing it into the tubs and containers.

Manufacturers are only able to put pictures of fruit on the label if the ice cream actually has fruit in it. So any ice cream marked 'strawberry-flavoured' for example, will have never seen a strawberry and will be artificially flavoured.

So there we have it - the bulk of the ice cream in that cornet you're holding is comprised of little more than vegetable fats and air. Even the flavour is fake, produced by a mix of who knows what chemicals. Nutrients? - forget it!

Farmed Salmon

Fish farming, also known as aquaculture, is the fastest growing form of food production in the world. 50 percent (70 percent for salmon) of the world's seafood is now produced this way.

Salmon is very popular and not just because of its unique flavour. As an oily fish, it also has health-giving properties due to its high content of omega-3 fatty acids. Salmon caught in the open seas is one of the most nutritious foods you can eat. The same, however, cannot be said of farmed salmon.

A study carried out in 2016 discovered that while farmed salmon are fatter than their wild cousins, they had half the level of omega-3 fats. This was thought to be due to the lower quality feed (consisting mainly of genetically modified grain and poultry litter) they are fed.

Farmed salmon are forced to live an unnatural life spent in inadequately sized enclosures. They are also exposed to pollutants such as dioxin and DDT, not to mention carcinogens. Salmon contaminated with these can cause a range of health issues.

To avoid eating farmed salmon, do not buy anything labelled 'Atlantic salmon' - this comes from fish farms. Also, be aware that virtually all salmon sold in restaurants and supermarkets is farmed. However, if you can find Alaskan salmon, buy it - it is actually illegal to farm Alaskan salmon.

Margarine

Once upon a time (and it wasn't that long ago) if you wanted something to spread on a slice of bread or to bake with, you used butter. It was cheap, tasty and good for you. Furthermore, people had been eating it for centuries without issue. Then cardiovascular disease began to raise its ugly head and pretty soon the so-called experts came to the erroneous conclusion that saturated fat was the cause of it all.

Sales of foods high in saturated fats like cheese, meat and, of course, butter, began to plummet. Desperate to find something to replace the cash cow that was butter, the food companies told their laboratories to concoct a replacement. The product they came up with looked like butter, smelled a bit like butter and tasted, well, a bit like butter. They called it margarine and told the world it was much healthier.

But of course it wasn't - it was actually a lot worse for us than butter. Scandalously, the manufacturers were only too well aware of this but did their utmost to convince us otherwise. It worked for a while but when the incidence of heart disease stubbornly continued to rise, the penny eventually dropped.

Why is margarine bad for us? Well, because the main ingredient is hydrogenated vegetable oils, aka trans fats. Amongst other things, they cause heart disease and stroke. The fact that margarine also contains synthetic colouring to disguise its grey, bland unappealing look maybe tells its own story!

More recently, in response to the criticism they have received, the manufacturers have tried to rescue the product by replacing the trans fats with palm oil. However, this is an oil rich in a type of fat that can also cause heart disease.

So it's back to square one. The fat in margarine, be it trans fats or palm oil, causes heart disease, stroke and other conditions. As to what all the chemicals in it do to us, well who knows? - if the manufacturers do, they're not saying!

So do yourself a big favour and don't eat this extremely unhealthy so-called food.

Peanuts

Peanuts originated in South America and were an important constituent in the diets of the Aztecs and other native Indian tribes. Today, they are an extremely popular snack food, as is a derivative - peanut butter.

As we have already seen, nuts in general are an extremely healthy food and peanuts, while not classed as a nut, are often thought of as such. However, while they may be very good for us in their natural state, by the time they arrive on the shop shelves, they are considerably less so.

Most peanuts are sold in packs and are coated in salt and vegetable oil. A large proportion of salt is a mineral called sodium and too much of it will raise your blood pressure. This increases the risk of cardiovascular disease and stroke. You can avoid this, though, by eating peanuts in the shell.

Peanut crops are heavily contaminated with pesticides, some of which are thought to be carcinogenic. Also, due to their soft skins, the nuts are susceptible to a fungus that releases a cancer-causing agent known as aflatoxin. This attacks the liver and is one of the most deadly food-borne toxins in existence.

Peanuts have a very high content of omega-6 fatty acid. This is important for us in a number of ways that include fighting inflammation, cognitive function and bone health. However, too much of it can actually be bad for us and increase the risk of getting common diseases, such as diabetes and Alzheimer's.

With regard to peanut butter, this is usually adulterated with palm oil or trans fats, plus salt and sugar for flavour. It will also be laced with the usual chemical preservatives.

Low-Fat Foods

Increasingly, people are becoming aware of just how precious their health really is and are now actively seeking ways to at least maintain, if not actually improve it. Currently, saturated fat is seen as being public enemy No 1 and the food companies, never slow to spot a new market, are busily selling us a range of low-fat products marketed as being healthy.

Walk down the aisles of any supermarket and your eyes will be assailed by shelves and shelves of low-fat this and low-fat that - biscuits, cakes, desserts, ready meals - all screaming at you, 'I'm healthy, eat me'.

Now, there's no disputing that these products are indeed low in fat. However, having taken out a major part of the food (as the saturated fat is), the companies have had to replace it with something else.

Until recently, they would have used trans fats for

this purpose. However, as they are having to scale back on the use of this type of fat, their solution is to instead use a blend of sugar, flour, thickeners, salt and chemical mixes of various kinds. This replaces the bulk and flavour lost by the removal of the fat.

Accordingly, most low-fat foods contain a lot more sugar than their full-fat equivalents - in many cases, several times as much. They also contain more modified starches, not to mention a range of chemical substances. The end result is food high in carbohydrates and calories, and actually anything but healthy! Don't fall for it.

Processed Meats

Meats that are processed include sausages, hot dogs, salami, bacon, ham, salted meat, corned beef, smoked meat, dried meat, beef jerky and tinned meat - there are many others as well.

Typically, the animals from which these meats are produced are raised in enclosures in much the same way that farmed fish are kept in pens. Not only do the poor animals live a short and wretched life but, as with the fish, they have an unnatural diet consisting largely of genetically modified grains.

Also, due to the unhygienic conditions in which they are compelled to live, the animals are given drugs - these include hormones and antibiotics. Furthermore, they are pumped full of various chemicals to not just preserve the meat but also give it colour and flavour.

Another issue with processed meats is the large amount of salt they contain. Years ago this was necessary in order to preserve meat but these days chemicals are used instead. The reason it is salted now is to add flavour. However, because of the large quantities of salt used, eating too much of these meats can cause hypertension, heart disease and some cancers - stomach and bowel cancer in particular.

If eaten very occasionally, processed meats won't do you any harm. Any more than that though, and you will be potentially exposing yourself to a range of illnesses and diseases. You'll also be supporting and furthering an industry that treats the animals in its care atrociously. I'll leave you to ponder the ethics of that!

Fruit Drinks
Of all the so-called health foods, fruit drinks must be at the top of the list of misrepresented products - the advertising and promotion blurb for them is just a massive lie. It's not hard to see why it works either.

Fruit is inherently healthy and people fondly imagine that all the food companies do is take a load of fruit, squeeze the juice out it, put it in cartons and then ship it off to the stores.

The reality, however, is different. The first problem with fruit juice is the large amount of sugar it contains. If you're eating an apple say, quite apart from its sugar content, you're also ingesting a lot of fibre. This fills you up and kills your appetite. Effectively, the fibre stops you eating too many apples thus making sure your intake of sugar is kept at a safe level. It also ensures the sugar is digested slowly at a rate the liver can handle.

Fruit drinks, however, don't contain any fibre, it's all been taken out. Consequently, a glass of it contains the sugar of not just one fruit, but several. One glass of apple juice contains the sugar of around eight apples!

Also, due to the lack of fibre, the rate at which it is digested is rapid. Accordingly, the body receives a large and sudden hit of sugar, which the liver cannot cope with. It uses what it can and converts the rest to fat.

One of the big selling points of fruit drinks is their supposedly high content of vitamins and other nutrients. This is true only to a degree, however, as the production process removes a large proportion of the nutrients. What's left, pound-for-pound, bears little relation to the nutritional content of whole fruit.

Another effect of the production process is that the

flavour, colour and odour of the fruit is largely removed. To make the juice look, taste and smell like it should, the sugary water that it essentially is, is enhanced with 'flavour packs' that are basically a cocktail of chemicals.

Calorie for calorie, fruit drinks are as bad for you as fizzy drinks, and my advice is to not drink them at all. They are a major contributor to the current obesity epidemic, plus, there is a confirmed link between them and tooth decay.

Much better by far to purchase a blender and make your own natural fruit drinks, the sugar content of which can be controlled.

Cereal

Just as with low-fat foods, supermarket shelves are packed with brightly coloured cereal boxes all proclaiming what a low sugar content they have, how much fibre they contain, what they are fortified with, etc, etc.

True to form, however, many of these claims are hugely exaggerated. Meanwhile, things the manufacturers would tell us about if they were genuinely concerned about our health, aren't mentioned at all.

Consider the way that cereals are manufactured. It's a highly mechanised process that starts with grain -

usually corn, wheat, rice or oats. This is cleaned, crushed and then pressure cooked. While the grain is cooking, various chemicals and fats are added. What rolls out the other end is an unappetising sludge devoid of shape, taste or smell.

Furthermore, because the outer layers of the grain have been removed during the processing, and the fact it's been subjected to very high temperatures, very little in the way of nutrients remains either.

The sludge is then dried and shaped. The last stage of the process is the adding of artificial flavouring, colouring, preservatives, sugar and nutrients. The latter enables the manufacturers to claim that the product has been 'fortified' with extra nutrients such as vitamins, iron and calcium.

However, the reality is that these so-called nutrients are synthetic, i.e. manufactured in a laboratory, and bear no relation to the real nutrients lost during the manufacturing process.

Then there is the fact that the grains used to make the cereals are almost always genetically modified. Health issues associated with GM foods include infertility, accelerated aging, faulty insulin regulation and problems with the gastrointestinal system and main organs.

Genetically Modified (GM) Food

Genetic modification is a laboratory procedure whereby genes from the DNA of one species are extracted and then forced into the genes of a different plant or animal. These extracted genes can come from bacteria, insects, viruses, animals or even humans.

Foods produced from, or using GM organisms, are referred to as genetically modified foods.

The benefits of genetic modification are that it improves crop yields by making plants naturally resistant to diseases, and also makes them more tolerant to herbicides. These benefits are purely economic - health-wise, there are none.

However, in years to come, it is forecast that genetic modification will be able to improve food's nutritional content, reduce its potential for creating allergies, and improve the efficiency of food production systems. GM foods will also be developed from microorganisms and animals unlike just from plants as they are now.

Is genetically modified food safe to eat though? Well, according to the scientific community the answer is yes. Predictably, the big corporations, who have a vested interest, say the same.

However, given that GM has only been around for about 30 years, no one can possibly know for sure. The jury is still out on its long term effects and, for that reason, I advise against it.

Also, as I have already mentioned, there is no reason to eat GM food at the moment - it offers no health benefits whatsoever. That being the case, why take the risk?

Organic Foods

The term 'organic food' refers to the product of a farming system that avoids the use of man-made fertilisers, pesticides, growth regulators and livestock feed additives. The system also prohibits irradiation and the use of genetically modified organisms (GMOs).

Basically, organic agriculture is about going back to the way farming was hundreds of years ago. It is a way of farming that is, to a large degree, dictated to, and controlled by, nature - not the other way round as happens with modern agricultural methods. As a result, the land and waterways are less polluted, wildlife can flourish and thrive, and the animals live in more pleasant, natural and humane conditions.

With the increasing focus on health, organic food is becoming increasingly popular. Many people, however, find it can be a very confusing subject. Are the benefits worth the premium prices charged? Is it really more nutritious than conventional food? Is organic food really better for the environment? What do all the labels mean? What, really, is the truth?

Lets take a look:

The Good
One of the most touted benefits of organic food is that it's exposed to fewer chemicals. In conventional farming,

the use of chemicals such as pesticides and fungicides are widespread. So many people will be surprised to learn that they are also widespread in organic farming.

There is, however, a difference. The pesticides used in organic farming are natural, as opposed to the synthetic pesticides used in conventional farming. While they are still toxic, the degree of toxicity is much less than with the synthetic pesticides. So, overall, the exposure to harmful chemicals is much less with organic food.

Organic food is much fresher than food grown conventionally as it doesn't contain preservatives to make it last longer, i.e. increase it's shelf life. Also, organic food is often produced on small farms that sell it locally - it doesn't need to be transported far and stored for long periods.

In most countries, organic crops don't contain genetically modified organisms (GMOs), and organic meat comes from animals raised on GMO-free farms.

Organic meat and milk is richer in omega-3 fats and certain minerals than from animals raised conventionally. As I have pointed out previously, these omega-3 fats provide us with a range of health benefits.

Organic farming is more environment-friendly due to the methods it employs. For example, its use of compost, manure and crop rotation. This helps to keep soil healthy and rich in organic matter, nutrients and microbial activity. It also uses much less energy - this is a very important factor these days.

Many people take the issue of animal welfare seriously. Organic farmers are legally obliged to do the same by providing their animals with access to the outdoors and allowing them to roam freely. They are also prohibited from using antibiotics and synthetic growth hormones. Furthermore, they must ensure their animals are fed 100 percent organic feed and provided with clean, cage-free living conditions.

Organic foods are generally considered to taste much better than conventionally produced foods. This is due to a higher mineral content and the fact that they are free of additives and chemicals.

The Bad
Cost - using chemicals and synthetic pesticides in conventional farming reduces the cost of production as they enable foods to be produced faster and more efficiently. Organic farms can't use these products and so inevitably, their rate of production is lower. Together with higher overheads, this makes organic products more expensive.

Organic foods are not treated with chemical preservatives, so they have a shorter shelf life than conventional foods do. This further adds to their cost.

Organic farming is big business and needs to sell its products. Exaggerated claims that it does this, that and the other are a favourite way of achieving this. One such claim is that organic food is far more nutritious than conventionally produced food.

However, there is no real evidence that this is the case. While organic food does have a higher content of *some* nutrients, it is definitely not *far more* nutritious.

Unfortunately, many organic farms don't take the issue of animal welfare as seriously as they would have us believe (and are supposedly obliged to by law). Yes, they let the chickens out of the cages but it may only be for a few minutes rather than the hours it should be.

All too often, the animals are forced to live in the same cramped, unpleasant conditions that conventionally farmed animals are. If they fall ill, they may not be given antibiotics because the farm would then lose its 'organic' status.

Animals on organic farms often have to endure the same cruelties, such as debeaking, castration and dehorning (and without painkillers!) - as animals on conventional farms do.

To Buy or Not to Buy

It's a fact that not all conventionally farmed foods are high in pesticides. Many people will still want to avoid them for other reasons - for example, their impact on the environment. But with regard to health, it is not always necessary to go for the more expensive organic versions.

The foods listed below are not high in pesticides for the simple reason they do not need to be:

- Asparagus
- Avocados
- Mushrooms
- Cabbages
- Sweet Corn
- Eggplants
- Kiwis
- Honeydew Melons
- Cantaloupes
- Mangoes
- Onions
- Papayas
- Pineapples
- Sweet Peas
- Sweet Potatoes
- Grapefruits
- Water Melons
- Cauliflowers

However, these foods are high in pesticides, so buying organic is the recommended option:

- Apples
- Spinach
- Apples
- Pears
- Celery
- Kale
- Squash
- Nectarines
- Peaches
- Spinach

- Tomatoes
- Bell Peppers
- Potatoes
- Strawberries
- Hot Peppers
- Grapes

How do you know if a food really is organic though? Well, in most countries organic foods are clearly labelled as such. In the USA and the EU, at least 95 percent of the ingredients in an organically labelled food product must be organically produced.

In some countries, the rules governing organic food labelling are ambiguous. For example, food with a low organic content may be labelled as 'made with organic ingredients'. It's true but deceptively so!

You should also be wary when buying organic foods from market traders and the like - very often they're anything but!

Juicing

Sales of juice extractors are going through the roof as more and more people find themselves tempted by all the hype being spread on the Internet and by various celebrities.

These machines extract the juice, and only the juice, from fruits and vegetables - all the pulp and fibre is removed. The end product is a thin watery liquid that contains all the nutrients the fruit or vegetable has to offer.

It certainly sounds healthy enough and does have some benefits. However, as we shall see, there are some definite downsides to juicing as well.

The Good

One obvious benefit is that it enables people who don't like a particular fruit or vegetable, and so would never eat it, to get the nutrients it offers.

Another is that by eliminating the starchy, and thus high in carbohydrates, part of the food, juicing can help people to lose weight.

Juicing provides an excellent way of ensuring that you get the recommended 'five a day' that virtually every health authority insists on these days. There is, actually, a lot of merit in this and having a juicer makes it very easy to do.

You are more likely to try a wider variety of fruit and vegetables. This increases the range of nutrients you take in and will undoubtedly have beneficial effects on your overall health.

The Bad

The most obvious disadvantage of juicing is the cost. Juicing is expensive when you compare it to eating whole fruits and vegetables. To start with, the juice extractors themselves are quite costly. Then there's the food - you'll need a lot more of it than if you were eating it whole. Whereas eating one or two apples would fill you up, getting a worthwhile amount of juice will need quite a few.

Juicing can make you ill. This is because raw food contains microbes, which can be the cause of a range of conditions such as food poisoning, vomiting, diarrhoea, e.coli, hepatitis and even kidney failure. For this reason, commercially produced juices and smoothies are put through a pasteurization process that kills all organisms that are potentially dangerous. Home-made versions are not!

Drinking vegetables is not the same as eating them. You may be getting the nutrients but you won't be getting the fibre that slows the speed at which they are digested. Health-wise, this is as important as the nutrients themselves.

Fibre is also essential for the promotion of beneficial bacteria in the digestive tract. These bacteria play an important role in preventing constipation and diseases of the gut, such as bowel cancer and inflammatory bowel disease. Fibre is also known to play a major role in keeping our immune systems healthy.

It's easy to overdo things and take in a concentrated dose of nutrients that your body simply isn't designed to handle. When this happens, the body will usually absorb what it needs and then excrete what's left. It doesn't always, however - some water-soluble vitamins taken in excess can cause problems. For example, too much vitamin B6 can cause nerve problems and excess vitamin C can cause kidney stones.

Problems also arise when just, or mainly, fruit is juiced. This can result in a drink that has far more sugar than is healthy. For example, juice five large oranges and you'll get a drink that contains about twenty teaspoons of sugar. Quite apart from all the health issues this can cause, it is very bad for your teeth and gums.

TIP - with some fruits and vegetables, many of the nutrients are actually in the skin, or just under it - avocados being a typical example. It's precisely this part that many people will discard during the preparation process. Don't make this mistake yourself.

Smoothies

As with juicing, making smoothies requires a machine; in this case one that blends all the ingredients into a mushy, pulpy liquid. The machines provide a quick and convenient way of getting nutrition.

The Good

Unlike with juicing, smoothie machines just pulp the fibre, they don't remove it. As a lot of a food's nutrients are in the fibre, this results in drinks that are healthier.

When compared to juicing, another benefit is cost. You don't need as much food to produce a smoothie as you do for a glass of juice.

Blending fruits and vegetables in the form of a smoothie is a quick and easy way to fuel your body. You can also add other types of food to enhance its nutrient content generally, or more specifically. As an example of the latter, adding nuts will give a smoothie a boost of protein.

Smoothies can be a lot more than just a drink. With a bit of thought and imagination, it is possible to come up with concoctions that are actually meal-substitutes. These can keep you going until lunch or whatever.

Smoothies make it easier to eat stuff that you don't like the taste of. All you have to do is blend it with something you do like the taste of.

The Bad

Smoothies are not, and never will be, as good for you as eating whole fruits and vegetables. There are several reasons for this. One is that during the blending process, the fibre is pulped and, inevitably, some is damaged. This means that the amount in the finished drink is not as much as would be gained from eating the fruit or vegetable whole.

Another is due to the process of oxidation (also an issue with juicing). As soon as the skin of a fruit or vegetable is broken, its flesh is exposed to light and air. This causes the nutrients in it to start breaking down almost immediately.

To demonstrate this, cut into an apple and you will see that the area around the cut very quickly turns brown - this is oxidation at work. So right from the word go, your smoothie is losing its nutritional value and, the longer you store it, the more it will lose.

Smoothies can be very high in both sugar and calories. It's very easy to get carried away when making these drinks and add things you really shouldn't, or simply just too much of them. One way to prevent this is to add leafy green vegetables that are generally quite tasteless. This will leave less room for the sugary stuff (and provide more nutrients as a bonus).

Smoothies can even be dangerous. This is due to the shape of the blending machine's cutting blades that makes them difficult to clean.

As a result, many people don't do it as well as they should with the result that the blades and the surrounding area become a breeding ground for harmful bacteria. These can cause food poisoning and diseases such as e.coli and salmonella.

Intermittent Fasting

Intermittent fasting is a scheduled eating plan in which food intake is restricted to a certain length of time. The most common way is to restrict eating to a window of about six to eight hours. This can be done daily, every other day or even weekly.

How Intermittent Fasting Works

When you are fasting intermittently, your body functions differently during the 'feasting' stage than it does during the 'fasting' stage. The food you eat during the feasting period is digested and the energy it contains is extracted into the blood stream. As it is in the blood, and thus immediately available, this is the energy your body will burn.

During the fasting period however, the opposite happens. As you haven't eaten for a long time, there is no surplus energy in your blood stream just waiting to be used. So when energy is needed, your body has to take it from the next available source - it's fat stores.

Typically, the fast times are between sixteen and eighteen hours - some people do it for longer periods such as thirty six hours and even several days. I don't advise this though, as it is taking the concept to extremes that really aren't necessary.

The way I do recommend is to simply stop eating breakfast, eat your lunch around midday and your dinner by 6.00 pm. Then eat nothing until lunch the following day and so on. By doing so, you'll be eating within a six hour window and fasting for eighteen hours.

If done correctly, intermittent fasting offers a range of benefits that include the following:

Weight Loss
The theory of intermittent fasting as an aid to weight loss is based on the fact that the body stores sugar as glycogen in the liver but only enough for six to eight hours. So assuming nothing else is eaten during this period, i.e. the glycogen store is not topped up, after six to eight hours it will all have been used up.

This compels the body to switch to the next available fuel - its stores of fat. Essentially, the process replicates what our ancestors were exposed to in terms of food availability.

Intermittent fasting compels you to eat less frequently. Unless you eat more when you do eat in order to compensate, your calorie intake will be less and you will lose weight - it's as simple as that!

Intermittent fasting also induces changes in the way certain hormones act. For example, HGH - human growth hormone. Intermittent fasting causes levels of these hormones to rise, one effect of which is to trigger the burning of fat. At the same time, it also helps build muscle.

Another effect of these hormonal changes is that the body's metabolic rate increases by up to 15 percent. This in turn leads to even more calories being burned and so weight being lost.

An interesting aspect of intermittent fasting as a means of losing weight is that a lot of the fat burned is from around the waist - traditionally the most difficult part of the body from which to lose fat.

Normalised Insulin Resistance
Insulin is a hormone produced by the pancreas and its purpose is to enable the body's cells to absorb glucose.

When the body becomes insulin resistant, its cells cannot absorb glucose as they should and so to compensate, it produces more and more insulin. Eventually, the pancreas can no longer produce enough of the hormone for the body's needs. The result of this is a sharp rise in blood sugar level.

Causes of insulin resistance include:

- being overweight or obese
- a diet high in carbohydrates

- a sedentary lifestyle
- high doses of steroids
- chronic stress

Ensuring none of these apply to you will eliminate, or at least considerably reduce, the risk of insulin resistance. Another method is intermittent fasting. Recent studies have demonstrated that it reduces both blood sugar levels and insulin by a considerable degree.

Reduced Effects of Aging on the Brain
Research shows that intermittent fasting can have a significant effect on the human brain. This works in two ways:

The first is that intermittent fasting causes the body to stop using glucose as an energy source and instead use fat. When it does this, the fat releases substances known as ketones. These are used by the body, the brain in particular, as an alternative fuel source. As ketones are a more efficient fuel than glucose, the brain receives a significant boost of energy.

The second is that ketones increase the number of mitochondria (minute organs that generate energy) in brain cells. This happens particularly in the hippocampus, a part of the brain that handles learning and memory. Cells in the hippocampus are known to degenerate when subjected to age-related brain diseases

146

such as Alzheimer's and Parkinson's Disease. This leads to cognitive impairment, loss of memory and more.

However, thanks to the increased amount of energy provided by the ketones, brain cells that would otherwise die are able to survive.

The takeaway here is that intermittent fasting is associated with improved motor coordination, learning response and a decrease in oxidative stress (oxidative stress is what we often consider normal age-related change). So intermittent fasting improves healthy aging of the brain and decreases the cognitive decline that is generally considered a normal part of the aging process.

Regeneration of the Immune System

Humans have a type of cell known as stem cells that can mutate into different types of cell. These stem cells stay dormant until they are activated by disease or an injury to body tissue.

When they are activated, they have the ability to generate a range of cell types from the originating organ, or even regenerate the entire original organ. In other words, stem cells provide the body with a way of repairing and renewing itself.

A related body function is known as mitophagy, the literal meaning of which is 'self eating'. This is a process

147

that enables the body to clean and detoxify itself by, quite literally, eating cells that are no longer needed or are damaged. The process is also thought to have a role in controlling the body's immunity system and inflammation.

However, mitophagy doesn't just happen - it has to be kick-started. The way to do it is by subjecting the body to an unusually high level of stress. There are three methods of doing this:

The first is by exercise. Working out actually damages your muscles by causing microscopic tears that the body then has to heal. This makes the muscles stronger than before, more resistant to further damage, and also builds new tissue. The more intense the exercise, the greater the benefit.

The second is by eating a ketogenic diet as discussed on pages 58-61. This forces the body to burn fat to fuel itself and enables people to lose body fat while retaining muscle.

The third is intermittent fasting. Although it wasn't always so, this is now an unnatural thing for us to do and our bodies find it a stressful experience as a result. When the body is in a 'fed' state, mitophagy is low. However, when in a 'fasted' state, the opposite applies - insulin levels drop and mitophagy increases.

Reduced Risk of Cardiovascular Disease

Triglycerides are a type of fat that is used to store excess energy from our diet. A high level of it is associated with cardiovascular disease and insulin resistance. Intermittent fasting is known to reduce the level of this type of fat significantly.

Reduced Levels of Inflammation

Inflammation is the immune system's response to damage or danger. This can be bacteria infecting a wound or a splinter piercing your finger, for example. It is not always helpful to the body though - with some types of disease the immune system actually attacks itself by mistake. Examples of this include Rheumatoid arthritis, Psoriasis and Crohn's disease. These are all chronic inflammatory diseases that can last for years, or even a lifetime, in varying degrees of severity.

A substance called Leukotriene B4 plays an important role in a number of cellular processes involved in inflammation. It is known that a diet high in fish oil decreases the production of Leukotriene B4. With this fact in mind, recent studies have been done to see if a reduction in calorie intake would also have a beneficial effect. The results have all shown that fasting, both intermittent and long-term, causes a decrease in the production of Leukotriene B4, and thus has an anti-inflammatory effect.

Do's and Don'ts of Intermittent Fasting

Intermittent fasting is straightforward enough. That said, there are a few things you need to be aware of before you start:

DON'T do it if you are pregnant, diabetic, have any underlying medical problems or are taking prescription drugs.

DO listen to your body. If you feel abnormal in any way, don't be a hero - stop immediately. In particular, heart palpitations, dizziness and weakness must not be ignored.

DON'T do strenuous exercise while fasting. Light stuff is fine, but it's best to avoid things like high-intensity cardiovascular exercise, especially if you're not used to it.

DO ensure you are drinking enough water. A large proportion of our water intake is from the foods we eat, so you will need to compensate by drinking more than you normally do.

DON'T fast intermittently if your usual diet comprises a lot of processed foods. Addressing the quality of your diet is crucial before you start fasting. Take a couple of weeks to slowly cut back on the refined carbohydrates, sugar and grains. Foods you should eat are vegetable carbohydrates, protein and healthy fats such as butter, eggs, cheese, avocados, coconut oil, olive oil and nuts.

DO work to a schedule by only eating in the same window. Working to a routine does make it easier to stick with.

DON'T give up! Half of the fasting period is when you're asleep. That just leaves eight hours or so. Drink water and tea whenever you start to waiver.

Part Four - The Processed Food Industry

I've mentioned the processed food industry a number of times so far and have yet to be complimentary. I'm now going to take a closer look at this monument to corporate greed and corruption and, in the process, show quite clearly just what a horror story the PFI really is.

It is no exaggeration to say that much of the food they con us into buying is, quite literally, nothing less than poison. This ranges in level of severity from merely making us feel a bit poorly to actually killing us. In-between, these foods cause diseases and conditions that ruin millions of people's lives.

Bereft of conscience, morality and lacking any scruples whatever, the PFI exists purely to make money - nothing else concerns it. Shockingly, the PFI's lies, deceit and complete disregard for its customers is all condoned by the very laws and lawmakers that are supposed to protect them.

How They Get Away With It

Given their way of doing business is sharp practice at best, and totally illegal at worst, you may well wonder how the big corporations that comprise the processed food industry manage to deceive their customers and disregard the laws that exist to protect those customers.

Secrecy is their main strategy. Very few people have any conception, either of what's in the processed food they eat, or of the ways the industry ensures they don't. Which is just the way the PFI like it. Make enquiries, as I have, and you hit a brick wall every time. Truly, this industry could be the blueprint for a country's secret service!

After a number of requests for interviews with various food corporations had been brusquely refused, I managed to trick my way into one by offering fake credentials. However, even though they thought they were talking with one of their own, I found they were still very guarded in what they said. What answers you do get from these people are phrased in bland corporate speak that gives as little away as possible.

Ask a company what's in a particular product and they simply refuse to tell you - commercial confidentiality is the usual excuse, i.e. we don't want our competitors to know! Ask to look around one of their factories and you'll get the old health and safety excuse, i.e. factories are dangerous places!

In reality, it's neither our health or competition they're worried about - their only concern is preventing us from finding out what they're doing.

Take a look at the websites of these companies and

you will quickly see that there is nothing remotely informative or illuminating. There'll be plenty of press releases, advertising, company statistics and so on, but no hard facts about what goes into their products.

Another favourite strategy is deception. Often, it doesn't take long for the public to become aware of suspect additives - E numbers being a typical example. Social media and the Internet ensure these suspicions spread quickly and sales of the product in question drop as a result.

The PFI's solution is to just replace the additive with something virtually identical but give it a different name - one that sounds reassuringly healthy. We'll see more on this tactic later.

When necessary, the PFI resorts to the oldest strategy of all - corruption. Most countries have food standards bodies and agencies to ensure the public is protected from food companies selling dangerous products. Having no intention of being dictated to by anyone, however, the PFI has two ways of dealing with these bodies.

The first is to have their own people on them and thus rig things in their favour. The second is to use their corporate power and financial muscle to simply buy their way out of trouble when necessary. This same method is also used to bribe government officials at the highest levels. Nothing is beyond the food processing industry.

Labelling

For years now, the PFI has relied on additives to give their bland, tasteless base products the flavours and colours destroyed by the industrial processing that produces them. Chemical-based preservatives increase shelf life, while binders, emulsifiers, thickeners, gelling agents, foaming agents, glazing agents and many more, are used to create texture and an appetizing appearance.

The public, meanwhile, has had little or no idea they've been doing this. It was only when the introduction of new rules compelled the PFI to list all a product's ingredients on the packaging that this changed.

Unable to do so honestly as it would kill sales, they have resorted to deceiving the public with a ploy that has been given the misnomer 'clean labelling'. This involves replacing all suspicious sounding ingredients on a product's packaging with ones that sound natural, i.e. not out of a chemistry lab - as many of them indeed are!

An example of clean labelling is an additive called oregano extract. This is commonly added to processed meats such as salami. However, it is not there to provide the meat with a fragrant aroma. It's there because it's a very effective preservative that reduces the rate at which the meat goes off. Previously, the manufacturer would have used a less than user-friendly sounding additive, such as butylhydroxyanisole - also known as E300-21. Oregano extract sounds much nicer!

Now you may ask what's so bad about using oregano as a preservative? - it's a natural herb after all with no chemical associations. The answer reveals the deception that lies behind the concept of clean labelling.

Forget any notion of a nice-smelling fresh herb being sprinkled into the meat. Oregano extract is a powder produced by an industrial process that uses chemical solvents to strip out all the smell and taste (and nutrients) from the oregano. It may sound much more appealing but, in reality, is little better than the chemical preservatives it has replaced.

Of course, a product's labelling can be used to deceive the public in other ways as well. For example, to persuade them that a product has been made in a traditional way by using phrases such as 'free of preservatives' and 'additive-free'.

Another ploy is to try and persuade the public that a product is a health food. To this end, phrases such as 'low-fat' are used.

Ingredients

Modern-day processed food is mass-produced by huge corporations operating out of factories that are every bit as industrial and mechanised as, say, a car factory. The production process is similar as well. They buy the ingredients (often unrecognisable as food) and then turn them into something that looks, feels, smells and tastes enough like food to fool the public.

These ingredients are supplied by smaller food companies that work in much the same way as the corporations they supply. Some provide the base ingredients for products, usually by taking healthy whole foods and processing much of the colour, taste, texture and smell out of them. They do this because uniformity is key in the processed food industry - every one of a batch of products has to be exactly the same. Needless to say, the food's nutrient value is refined out as well.

Other companies specialise in additives that put the colour, taste, texture and smell back into the sludge the industrialised processing produces. I take a closer look at what's involved in this on pages 162-168.

These supply manufacturers are essentially an industry within an industry. And it's one that the general public knows virtually nothing about and will rarely, if ever, come into contact with. They market their products to the big corporations by means of food trade exhibitions that are strictly invitation only - the general public are *not* welcome.

This paranoid need for secrecy from all sides of the industry is as instructive as anything with regard to the quality and safety of the food they produce and sell.

Freshness
Virtually all supermarkets these days have 'in-store bakeries'. Walk past one and you will see rows of crispy looking loaves and smell the enticing aroma of newly baked bread. At the rear, you'll see large stainless steel ovens and staff busily taking out the freshly baked loaves and putting them on the shelves - it's all very convincing.

However, it's a setup and the customers are being conned. What they're actually buying is bread made somewhere else and which has then been frozen - probably for months. The supermarket shoves it in an oven, warms it up and then presents it to the customer as freshly made bread - it's actually just the opposite!

It's not just bread either. All dough-based foods such as

cakes, doughnuts, pastries, croissants, and so on are given the same treatment. Most high street bakeries and delicatessens work in exactly the same way.

Furthermore, because these products have been manufactured with no intention of being sold immediately, they are also adulterated with the usual array of chemical preservatives.

Continue your walk around the supermarket and you will come across the fresh fish counter. Here, you will see all manner of fish species enticingly laid out on beds of ice. As with the 'bakery', the setup is designed to create the impression of freshly caught fish. Once again, though, it's a con.

If you're very lucky, you may get some fish that actually is fresh. The reality, though, is you're much more likely to end up with something that is days old - and maybe even on the point of going rotten.

A recent article in a British newspaper described how a reporter observed fish from several English supermarkets being tested. Of the twelve samples, four failed to meet even the minimum level of acceptability (ten days since being caught). Basically, they were on the verge of rotting. Six were on the borderline. Shockingly, only two samples out of the twelve were found to score above it.

Perception

As we have just seen, whether the food they sell is fresh or not is immaterial to the PFI. Their only concern is that the food *looks* fresh and appetizing - it's a matter of perception. If it doesn't look good, people won't buy it.

However, the tricky bit for them is that not only does it have to look good, it has to *stay* looking good - and for as long as possible. This is where we encounter food preservatives. As with all additives, these are substances that either contain chemical compounds not found in natural foods, are chemically enhanced or are produced by chemical processes.

Their sole purpose is to keep food looking good long after it should do - a function that is of prime importance to the PFI. The actual quality of the food is secondary - nutritionally, it's of no importance to the PFI whatsoever.

Aware of the growing awareness and dislike of chemical additives, the PFI is continually on the lookout for new ways to deceive the public. A method they have recently begun using is a food packaging system known as Modified Air Packaging (MAP). This works by replacing the air in packaged food with an optimal blend of oxygen, carbon dioxide and nitrogen.

Without going into the details, it keeps food looking much fresher than it actually is - meat stays red, cheese doesn't go mouldy, etc, etc. The shelf life of food packaged in this way can be doubled - great for the PFI but not so great for the consumer who is buying food that can, quite literally, be weeks old.

Who on earth wants to be eating three-week old fish? What's more, as soon as the MAP packaged product is opened, it rapidly assumes the state it would naturally be in at such an age - limp, discoloured and with a bad taste. It doesn't matter to the PFI though - it's made another sale.

The 'edible film' con is another deception. This is a chemical substance that coats food with an edible film that is invisible, odourless and tasteless. The purpose of the film is to keep the food looking fresh and it works by keeping air away from it. The person eating the food has no idea they are eating something that could well be weeks old, nor that they are also eating a laboratory-inspired chemical cocktail.

Yet another technique employed by the PFI in its eternal quest for 'perceived freshness' is the use of enzymes. This is potentially quite scary stuff as it uses genetic modification techniques.

While nobody can say it is dangerous with any degree

of certainty, nor can anyone say it isn't? Do you want to be the one who finds out?

What these techniques (and others still in the pipeline) do is blur the boundaries. Nobody in their right mind would eat a chicken more than a couple of days old. The processed food industry, however, has no trouble in getting us to eat chicken that is much older because we *perceive* it as being fresh.

Taste

If the perceived freshness of a product ranks number one on the PFI's scale of importance, flavour runs it a close second. Having conned a customer into buying something that looks good, it then has to taste fairly good as well. If it doesn't, a repeat sale isn't likely.

The positively brutal techniques employed in industrial food processing - heat, centrifugation, deodorising, sterilisation and pasteurisation to name just some - inevitably results in loss of taste. So it has to be put back into the soggy, tasteless gunk that comes out the other side of the production line.

To this end, there is another range of additives known as flavourings - currently, there are some three thousand of them. They aren't there just to add flavour, however. The manufacturing process imparts unpleasant smells and flavours of its own, often from chemical solvents and contaminants, such as heavy metals. To deal with these, dual-role flavourings have come into being - not only do they provide the desired flavour, they also mask unwanted ones.

Another reason flavourings are so important to the PFI is that they are a lot cheaper than the real thing. For example, an orange flavouring additive costs much less than real oranges.

For the PFI therefore, the use of flavouring additives is a no-brainer. The consumer, though, may see it rather differently. No matter how hard their makers try, it's a fact that no artificial flavouring will ever taste as good as the real thing.

Older people who have been brought up with unprocessed food, and so have a benchmark, will immediately taste the difference between lemon squash made with lemons, and artificially flavoured lemon squash. Younger people, most of whom have never tried the real thing, won't.

More important than the unnatural taste left by these flavouring additives, however, is the fact that many of them are positively dangerous to our health. For example, solvents such as butane and propane are used in the production process, and it is a fact that some remain in the finished product. The PFI's stance on this is that the amounts involved are so minute that they pose no risk to our health.

If that's true, how do they explain away the fact that workers in factories producing crisps, pretzels and the like, have a much increased risk of respiratory diseases due to inhaling the flavouring additives. This being the case, what do they do to us when we eat them?

Then we have sugar, the most common additive of all. This substance is without doubt the most dangerous food known to man and yet the PFI puts it into everything. Just one of the many reasons they do so is in response to the current 'fat is bad' mantra.

Jolted into action by falling sales, the PFI has had to drastically cut the amount of fat in its products. And as most of the flavour in food comes from the fat, they have had to find something to replace it with. Sugar is their chosen option. However, as they were already using plenty of it, this has resulted in virtually all processed food being positively rammed with the stuff.

For example, one can of soup can contain five teaspoons of sugar, a can of soda up to nine teaspoons, a bottle of cooking sauce up to ten teaspoons. It's also the reason that foods marketed as being 'low fat' and 'healthy' are often anything but.

The problem with this high intake of sugar (particularly

the refined fructose favoured by the PFI) is the fact that the liver has a limited capacity to absorb and use it. We can actually only metabolize about six teaspoons of sugar per day - anything over and above is turned into fat. When you consider that the average westerner consumes about twenty teaspoons a day, the reason for the current obesity epidemic becomes clear.

As I have pointed out repeatedly, excess weight leads to a number of chronic metabolic diseases, such as type 2 diabetes, cardiovascular disease, high blood pressure, dementia and cancer. The PFI is well aware of all this but couldn't care less.

A particularly underhand trick they use is to put caffeine and salt in soft drinks. Caffeine is a diuretic that makes us urinate, and salt makes us thirsty - the two, in combination, keep us feeling unnaturally thirsty and so needing to buy more. To hide the taste of the salt, the PFI turns to its old standby - sugar - copious amounts of it!

They also go to enormous lengths to conceal the amount of sugar they use. The simplest is just giving it a different name - there are over sixty alternative names for sugar.

Another method takes advantage of the fact that ingredients are listed by weight on the packaging with the main ingredients listed first. This means that the more of something there is in a food, the higher up on the list it appears. To make their products appear healthier, they use small amounts of three or four different types of sugar in them - these small amounts add up to a large amount, though!

Texture

Another attribute that's extremely important to the PFI is texture. The food must not only look and taste good, it must *feel* good as well. This is as important a factor as any in convincing people that what they're eating is proper food. Unfortunately for the PFI, the processing procedures churn out food that tends to be somewhat lacking in this respect.

Once again, food additives come to the rescue - one of the main ones here being starch. Cheap, tasteless, odour-free, a neutral-white in colour and bulky, starch has little nutritional content and so offers virtually nothing to the consumer.

To the PFI, however, it is quite literally worth its weight in gold, due to the myriad uses it can be put to. It gives texture and bulk to bread, it adds crunch to biscuits, it makes chips crispy, it adds creaminess to mayonnaise, plus a hundred and one other things.

Needless to say this isn't a simple starch, such as

the cornflour commonly used in households up and down the land. No, the PFI have their own versions, called 'modified starches', that bear little resemblance to the household variety. Production methods for these starches include treatment with enzymes, acid, chemicals such as sodium and potassium hydroxide, and even electrical charging.

Predictably, the PFI claims modified starches are safe to eat but, given the fact they refuse to give exact details of how they make them, these claims have to be regarded with a degree of suspicion.

However, regardless of whether they are safe to eat or not, it is indisputable that these modified starches cheat the customer. This is because the PFI use them as a substitute for more expensive ingredients such as oils, eggs, cheese and butter.

This reduces their costs considerably, which wouldn't be so bad if some of it was passed on to the consumer. Needless to say, it never is. Furthermore, these modified starches, processed as they are, are totally devoid of any nutritional content. So in far too many cases, consumers are getting little or nothing for their money.

A final kick-in-the-teeth is the fact that starch has a high carbohydrate content. This means that not only is food that contains it low in nutrients, it's high in calories. So, being a main ingredient in virtually all processed food, starch contributes highly to the obesity levels that are rocketing all over the world.

We now come to the PFI's second favourite additive - water, and for the same reasons. This liquid is cheap and also an ideal bulking agent for making food portions look bigger than they actually are. This is very handy with more expensive foods like meat and seafood.

However, there is an inherent problem with getting meat and fish to absorb water. With meat that has been minced, such as sausages, meatballs and burgers, it's easy enough. But with solid pieces - ham, steak, chicken breasts, prawns, etc, special equipment is needed. This is a machine through which the meat is passed, and which pierces the meat with rows of fine needles that inject water into its tissues.

Meat treated in this way can be anything up to fifty percent water. Furthermore, this is PFI water we're talking about - not nice, clean tap water. Known in the trade as brine, this is water that has been treated with chemicals to give it 'added properties'. This brine is used to provide texture and feel to a range of processed foods, as well as for bulking.

Packaging
All processed food is packaged. It's not done for the

customers benefit but because it has to be, and for several reasons:

The first is marketing. Look at the picture on a box showing the ready-made meal it contains and you will see a professionally photographed image portraying tender cuts of meat and crisp, perfectly cooked vegetables. Open the box and you will almost certainly see something rather different!

Packaging provides another way of extending shelf life. For example, the inside of tin cans are commonly lined with epoxy resins (as used in glues) to stop the metal reacting with the can's contents. Displayed meats are placed on chemically-treated mats that absorb blood - for use with fruit, these same mats can be supplied treated with fungicides. Clear plastic containers have a chemical coating on the inside to stop them 'fogging up'.

Thousands, quite literally, of toxic chemicals are used in the packaging of processed foods. These include carbon monoxide, ammonia, paraffin and formaldehyde, to name just some. Many are known to be the cause of serious health problems. Just one example of this is a group of chemicals called phthalates. These are used to make the type of plastic found in fast food containers such as pizza boxes.

A recent study has shown that people who eat this type of food regularly have dangerous levels of phthalates in their body. Take it from me - these chemicals are something you definitely don't want in your system!

When pressed on this issue, the PFI's response is depressingly familiar. There's no need to worry, they say, as the quantities of chemicals used are so infinitesimal, they can't possibly have any ill effects.

As the one at the sharp end, however, you may wonder at the cumulative effects of long-term intake of these substances.

Part Five - Lose Weight Sensibly

I am shortly going to present you with a diet plan that's guaranteed to not only make you lose weight, but to lose it in a healthy and sustainable way. To understand the rationale behind this diet plan, it is necessary to first take a look at the foods we have been eating over the years, why we have been eating them and what they have done to us.

The story starts not that long ago - we're only going back to the first half of the 1900's. This was a volatile time in world history, what with the two world wars, the Russian civil war, the Afghan civil war and the Mexican revolution. There were plenty of lesser conflicts as well.

Food would have been scarce anyway because the methods used in agriculture and farming were basic and inefficient. The various wars made it even scarcer. However, although it may not have seemed so at the time, this was not necessarily a bad thing for some.

With food limited, people who would perhaps have over-eaten and become overweight, or even obese, simply weren't able to do so. As a result, the incidence of heart disease and strokes was low.

The end of the second world war saw things improve rapidly. Industry and farming became increasingly mechanised, and hence efficient. Chemical pesticides and new types of fertilisers were developed that enabled farmers to vastly increase crop yields. Within a very short while, food shortages in the western world were a thing of the past.

The foods commonly eaten at this time were high in saturated animal fat - red meat, cheese, butter, full-fat milk, lard and cream. They were rich in nutrients and also nice to eat. However, food wasn't the only thing that was plentiful - cardiovascular diseases were now as well.

In fact, by the late 1950's, heart disease was pandemic in the USA and rapidly becoming so in countries such as Australia, New Zealand and Great Britain. In an attempt to discover why, government agencies were commissioned to investigate and find solutions. One of these studies - the Seven Countries Study - was conducted in 1958 by a scientist called Ancel Keys. This focused on the link between diet and cardiovascular disease in different countries.

The study concluded that the countries where people ate the most saturated fat had the highest rates of heart disease - the connection seemed obvious. However, for some reason, Keys ignored a number of contradictory facts.

One was that in some of the countries, like Holland and Norway, fat consumption was high but rates of heart disease were low. But in other countries, such as Chile, fat consumption was low but the rates of heart disease were high. Basically, Keys disregarded anything that didn't support his theory.

For some reason though, the American Heart Association allowed itself to be convinced by Keys, thus giving credence to the flawed study. Massive exposure in the media followed and, very quickly, the demonisation of saturated fat began.

Suddenly, it was all 'fat and cholesterol are bad for you' and 'carbohydrates from fruits, vegetables and grains are good'. This was the beginning of the obesity epidemic currently sweeping around the globe.

If people had stuck to eating mostly fruit and vegetables there wouldn't have been a problem. Not only is the carbohydrate content of both these food groups much less than that of grains, it is also digested by the body at a much lower rate thanks to their high fibre content.

Unfortunately, they didn't. Instead, they latched on to carbohydrate-rich grains. Most foods produced from wheat, barley, rye, oats, etc, go through an industrial process that removes virtually all their fibre, vitamins

173

and minerals. While they provide energy in the form of calories, they offer very little in the way of nutrition - they are basically just empty calories.

The other problem with them is that they are quickly and easily digested by the body - often in as little as two hours - a process that should take between six and eight hours! Because the body turns carbohydrates into glucose (sugar), the result is a rapid increase in both blood sugar level and insulin. After an hour or two, the sugar level will drop back and, in so doing, stimulate parts of the brain associated with reward and craving. These signals create a craving for more food and are a known cause of over-eating.

Now, if the person eating the carbohydrate is active to a sufficient enough degree, the body will use the glucose for fuel and simply burn it off. However, if not, the glucose won't be used and the body will instead store it as fat for use in emergencies such as famine - just what nature has programmed it to do.

Now, couple the above with the following:

Firstly, people lead sedentary lifestyles these days. Indeed, they spend most of their time sitting down. They sit in their offices at work, they sit in buses, cars and trains, they sit at the movies, they sit on the beach and they spend their evenings sitting in front of the

TV. Much of the time they're doing this sitting, they are eating and drinking and, therefore, taking in shed-loads of calories that their bodies simply don't need. The inevitable consequence is that they put on weight.

Secondly, it is a fact that many of the most popular foods and drinks on the planet consist mainly of carbohydrates, i.e. bread, cakes, rice, biscuits, pasta, pizzas, pastries, fruit drinks, sports drinks, etc. These are all naturally very high in calories, a fact that is compounded by the food manufacturers adding large amounts of refined sugar to make them more palatable. This makes these already fattening foods even more fattening.

Thirdly, regardless of what they are consuming, people these days are simply consuming far too much. It's understandable enough as eating and drinking are activities that we all enjoy; many of us however, are overdoing it. Another factor in this is the ready availability of food these days - if you have the money, you can have as much of it as you want, when you want.

The way we live our lives has had an effect as well. Years ago, eating was largely restricted to set mealtimes of breakfast, lunch and dinner. Now, with the instant availability of processed foods, people snack at all hours of the day and night, as well as eating at mealtimes.

This last point takes us back to the processed food industry which is so vast these days that it basically rules the world. As a result, their high-carbohydrate foods are everywhere - restaurants, supermarkets, shops, bus stations, airports - you name it and processed food will be there. It's so ubiquitous, in fact, that many people just don't bother cooking any more.

As I have already shown, the processed food industry is also an extremely dishonest one and packs its products with vast amounts of sugar, the presence of which it tries to conceal with sneaky product labelling. Because of this, many people are completely unaware of the horrifically high calorific content of the foods they are consuming.

And so to the situation as it is today. Since the 1980's, the number of overweight and obese adults in the developed world has quadrupled to around one billion. One in three adults is overweight. In western countries, such as the USA and the UK, the situation is even worse as two-thirds of adults are overweight. Of these, one in three is considered to be obese, and one in twenty is considered to be extremely obese. With regard to children and adolescents, the situation is not much better.

These people all have a much higher risk of cardiovascular diseases, such as heart attacks and strokes, which are now the leading causes of premature death in the world. They are also much more likely to get type 2 diabetes, high blood pressure, non-alcoholic fatty liver disease and osteoarthritis, not to mention cancers such as breast, colon, endometrial and kidney.

As I have pointed out, there are several factors at play here, such as sedentary lifestyles and the over-abundance of food. However, the main one is the fact that refined carbohydrates are a highly fattening food and, of these, the worst is sugar.

Therefore, the Eat For Life Diet that I recommend in this book is based on eating foods that either don't contain any carbohydrates or are very low in them. Merely cutting out sugar in its most obvious forms is not enough. You need to remember that your body converts all the carbohydrates you eat to sugar in the form of glucose - so, those carbs have to go!

While the diet eliminates a lot of the foods people have become accustomed to over the years and will therefore miss enormously at the beginning of it, the hard fact remains that these foods are basically empty calories that provide little or no nutrition.

They are also the foods that make people put on weight

- that's the bottom line!

What the diet does permit is a range of more natural foods that provide all the nutrients needed to fuel the body and keep it operating at it's maximum capacity. At the same time, the vastly reduced intake of carbohydrates means it is not constantly making the glucose sugar that invariably leads to the creation of body fat. Not only will it make you feel younger, it may even make you look younger!

The foods we are talking here are non-starchy vegetables, low-sugar fruits, nuts and seeds, fish, meat, eggs, spices, herbs, full-fat dairy products and some types of vegetable oil. With the exception of the vegetables, herbs, fruits and spices, they all contain high amounts of healthy fats.

To people raised on the old belief that eating fat makes you fat, this may make the diet sound contradictory but it's not. All the evidence now actually indicates the opposite - eating fat is good for you (and not fattening) as long as you eat the right type and in the right quantities.

The diet is also adaptable - it can be tweaked to suit your requirements. If it's rapid weight loss you want, the diet in its most extreme form will deliver weight loss in the region of half a pound a day. Combine it with intermittent fasting as I describe on pages 143-151 and you will lose even more.

At the other end of the scale, for those of you who are already at the right weight and just want to eat a healthy diet as a lifestyle choice, the Eat For Life Diet can, again, be the one to follow. In this case, instead of virtually no carbohydrates, it's quite possible to introduce a limited range of them. Remember, there are many carbohydrate-rich foods that are actually good for you. These include fruits, legumes such as lentils, beans and peas, and whole grains such as oats, quinoa and brown rice.

Not only do these foods increase the options available to you and so make the diet more varied and easier to persevere with, they provide a vital nutritional resource - fibre. You can even eat some carbohydrates that aren't particularly good for you - bread being a typical example.

The big no-no on the Eat For Life Diet is processed food. Basically, anything that comes in a box, packet or tin is processed to one degree or another. The nutritional value of this type of food is usually very poor. Plus, of course, it is invariably packed with carbs and hence calories.

What You Can and Cannot Eat

In Part Two we looked at the most popular diet plans out there. While they all have their pros and cons, none of them in my opinion are as good as they could be. For example, the Atkins and Ducan diets that restrict fibre intake in the early stages to a level that's low enough to be potentially dangerous.

A lot of them try to make you lose weight at a rate that is not good for you. To achieve this, these diets are extreme - in some cases, they forbid entire classes of food. So not only can they actually be bad for you, they can also be difficult to persevere with.

The diet that I advocate - the Eat For Life Diet - is different in a number of ways. Firstly, and unlike other diets, it is healthy and includes *all* the nutrients your body needs to keep firing on all cylinders. This is in stark contrast to some that actually do the opposite!

Secondly, while not designed to be a weight-loss diet as such, it is a fact that overweight people who follow it will lose weight as sure as night follows day. However, unlike with most other diets, the weight loss will be slow, steady, easily sustainable and, ultimately, much healthier.

Please note that the Eat For Life Diet is just part of what you need to do to get your body as fit and healthy as possible. The other part is exercise and this is every bit as important as the foods you eat and don't eat. That's another story though.

So, lets take a look at the foods you can and cannot eat on this diet.

Meat

White meat such as chicken is the favoured option as it contains less calories than red meat. This is due to its lower fat content. If you prefer red meat though, you need to choose carefully. Go for leaner cuts and trim off as much of the fat as you can.

Of the red meats, beef is the highest in calories with pork and lamb having slightly less. The red meat with the least amount of calories is game animals, such as deer, elk, rabbits, etc.

As regards processed meat, this must be given a wide berth - the processing leaves all types high in calories. The worst are the sausages, such as salami, hot dogs, bologna and chipolata. Not only are they padded out with highly fattening starches, they contain unhealthy additives.

Seafood

As we have already seen, nutrition-wise, there is little to choose between red/white meat and seafood. However, seafood has the edge with regard to it's fat content which is much less. As low fat means low calories, this makes seafood an extremely good option for the dieter.

There are many different types though - which ones do you go for? Unsurprisingly, the answer is the species with the least fat content; namely, cod, flounder, sole, hake, haddock, pollock and shellfish.

The species with the highest amount of fat, and so the highest calories, are the oily fish like herring, mackerel, sardines and salmon.

Note that with most fish species, the colour of the flesh indicates their fat content. The leanest species have a white or light colour and the fattier species usually have a darker colour.

Luckily, the low-calorie fish also happen to be the ones least affected by mercury and other sea contaminants.

Dairy Produce

Lets start with milk. The skimmed type, from which all the cream has been removed, is the lowest in calories. It is, however, tasteless - little more than water. If you can stomach the stuff, fine; if not, the next best option, and the one I recommend, is semi-skimmed milk.

While it may have more calories, it does at least have some flavour and nutritional content. Full-fat and raw milk should be avoided when on a weight-loss diet.

Moving on to cheese, this is, in general, a high calorie food that is not the best thing to be eating when trying to lose weight. With this in mind, you may be tempted by the low-fat cheeses on the supermarket shelves. Take my advice and give these a miss. As I've already mentioned, virtually all foods labelled as 'low-fat' are the processed food industry's attempt to cash in on the current trend for healthy eating. While foods given this label may indeed be low in fat, don't think for a minute they will also be low in calories - they won't!

However, one cheese in particular is naturally low in calories and so can be incorporated into a weight-loss diet. This is cottage cheese which has only 98 calories per 100g. At the other end of the scale are the hard cheeses such as stilton, cheddar and parmesan - all over 400 calories per 100gm and definitely to be avoided.

The situation with butter is largely the same as with cheese. It is simply too high in calories to be part of a weight-loss diet. There are products marketed as low-fat butter but these are usually spreads made with vegetable oils and margarine. As with low-fat cheeses, steer well clear.

Another very popular dairy food is yoghurt. Is it ok in a weight-loss diet though? Well, there's no question that the fruit yoghurts are high in calories, typically in the region of 250 calories per carton. Plain yoghurts on the other hand, of which Greek is an example, only have about 150 calories in a carton - much better. Once again, give the low-fat versions a miss - many of these contain alarming amounts of sugar.

Nuts

As we have already seen, nuts are extremely nutritious and offer vitamins, minerals, fibre and protein. They also have a lot of fat though, which gives them a high calorie count. On the face of it, this would seem to make them one of the last things to include in a weight-loss diet.

However, this isn't the case. There's plenty of evidence to show that dieters who eat a small quantity of nuts are more likely to stick to their diets. This is because the fat and fibre content of the nuts is extremely satiating and, as a result, they are not as hungry and, ultimately, eat less.

The key to it is portion control. All you need to eat is about one ounce of nuts per day - this equates to just one handful. With almonds, brazils, cashews, pistachios and walnuts, this will be about 170 calories. Peanuts have the lowest calories - 150, while pecans and macadamias are the highest at about 200 calories.

Vegetables

Vegetables are the dieter's best friend. Very low in calories so you can eat as much of them as you like and, at the same time, high in satiating fibre. Really, what more could you ask for?

First on your diet plan should be leafy greens such as kale and spinach. They are incredibly nutritious and very high in vitamins, minerals and antioxidants.

Next are the cruciferous vegetables like broccoli, cauliflower, brussels sprouts and cabbage. You should also eat peppers - hot peppers like chilli particularly. They contain a substance called capsaicin, which has been shown to help reduce appetite and increase the body's ability to burn fat.

The vegetables you don't want be eating are the root varieties - carrots, potatoes, parsnips, etc. These contain more starch and so are higher in calories.

Fruit

Fruits of all types are very good for us. They do, however, have an inherent problem - they all contain sugar to one degree or another. Some have a lot more than others and so can be quite high in calories.

The key to including fruit in a diet plan, therefore, is knowing which ones to avoid.

In the list of fruits that follow, the figures given are the calorie content in 100 grams of fruit.

The fruits with the lowest calorie count are: strawberries 33, honeydew melon 36, peaches 39, blackberries 43, nectarines 44, cranberries 46 and oranges 47

Fruits with a medium calorie count are: apricots 48, cherries 50, pineapples 50, apples 52, raspberries 53, tangerines 53, pears 57 and blueberries 57

The fruits with the highest calorie count are: mangoes 60, kiwifruit 61, grapes 67, guavas 68, bananas 89, figs 107 and dates 280

Be aware that dried fruits like raisins, sultanas, prunes, figs and dates have the highest sugar count of all, and most definitely should not be part of a weight-loss diet.

The nutrients in fruit are simply too good to miss out on, even when dieting. Accordingly, I recommend that the low calorie fruits should be part of your diet. The relatively small amount of sugar they contain is nothing to worry about.

Carbohydrates

Foods made from refined carbs are not worth eating - the nutrients have been stripped out, they're starchy, full of sugar and additives are needed to make them palatable.

However, this doesn't apply to carbohydrates left in their natural state. The main thing these offer to the dieter is fibre. As with the fibre in nuts and vegetables, this is filling and so acts as a powerful appetite suppressant. Accordingly, diets that include them are easier to adhere to.

It is a fact that fruits, vegetables and nuts all contain carbohydrates, and a diet rich in these foods will provide everything you need in this respect. However, you may have reasons of your own for limiting your consumption of them or indeed, not wanting to eat them at all.

If this is the case, the following carb-rich foods will be the perfect substitute. The ones we're talking about are legumes (lentils, beans and peas), whole-wheat pasta, oatmeal, whole-wheat bread and brown rice. Another good reason for including them in your diet is to add variety. Just remember they are quite starchy and so should be consumed in small amounts.

Liquids
With regard to what you can drink on a weight loss diet, there's only one contender really and that's water - lots of it. It's absolutely the best thing you can drink.

The worst, as we've seen, are soft drinks, juice drinks,

sports & energy drinks and alcohol.

Very few people, though, are going to stick rigidly to water and nothing else. Nor is there any need to. Smoothies, which we looked at on pages 140-142, provide a very good alternative. Just remember to leave out ingredients high in calories.

The most popular drink in the world next to water is tea. When flavourings and additives are added, such as sugar, milk, herb extracts, oils, etc, its calorific content goes up. Taken by itself, however, it is virtually calorie-free and can be drunk in any amount. In this form, it should be part of any diet.

Vegetable juices are another good option. These require a juicing machine as we saw on pages 134-139. Just don't over-do it - too much of a concentrated dose of vegetable nutrients isn't recommended.

Currently very popular is coconut water. This is the clear liquid found inside a green coconut. It's a healthy drink that has plenty of nutrients. It is also relatively low in calories and so can be taken in reasonable quantities. Just remember not to confuse it with coconut milk. Higher in fat and calories, a cup of coconut milk is about 550 calories compared to about 50 calories in a cup of coconut water.

The fruit drinks and squashes available in the shops all

have an extremely high sugar content and so have no place in any diet. However, there's no reason dieters can't make their own - it's just fruit squeezed into water after all. By doing so, they can adjust the amount of fruit and, hence sugar, it contains.

Lastly, there is alcohol. There's no question it shouldn't be drunk at all, never mind on a diet. However, it is a fact that many people can't get through life without it (author included). So, for these people, the best options are light beers, wine (both red and white) and neat spirits.

Don't imbibe any alcoholic drinks that contain mixers - this is where the calories come from. Sweetened drinks like cider are strictly taboo as well. Never, ever, go near the frozen alcoholic drinks you see in the supermarkets - these are liquid sugar!

Be aware that the calories in alcoholic drinks is not just down to the sugar they contain - their carb content is also a factor. Beer is a good example of this - virtually no sugar but, thanks to the carbohydrate content, quite high in calories.

The Eat For Life Diet

In Part Two we looked at the most popular diet plans out there. While they all have their pros and cons, none of them, in my opinion, are as good as they could be. For example, the Atkins and Ducan diets that restrict fibre intake in the early stages to a level that's low enough to be potentially dangerous.

A lot of them try to make you lose weight at a rate that is not good for you. To achieve this, these diets are extreme - in some cases, they forbid entire classes of food. So not only can they actually be bad for you, they can also be difficult to persevere with.

The diet that I advocate - the Eat For Life Diet - takes a different approach Firstly, and unlike other diets, it is healthy and includes *all* the nutrients your body needs to keep firing on all cylinders. This is in stark contrast to some that actually do the opposite!

It is low in calories but not ridiculously so. As a result, weight loss will be at a sensible rate. Not only is this healthier, it makes the weight loss more sustainable.

The plan is much more than just a way of losing weight. It is a way of eating that should be followed for life and will enhance and extend the life of everyone who embraces it. So, starting with breakfast, lets get to it.

Breakfast Recipes

Mushroom Quiche

The secret of this quiche is that it doesn't contain any pastry, i.e. carbohydrates.

Serves 4   **Prep time 15m**   **Cook time 30m**

300g mushrooms, coarsely chopped
1 onion, finely chopped
50g butter
2 tbsp dried breadcrumbs
2 tbsp parmesan cheese, grated
1/4 tsp black pepper, ground
100g cheddar cheese, grated
200g cream cheese
4 eggs
150g cooked ham or bacon, diced

In a medium pan, sauté the mushrooms and onion in the butter until just tender - about 5 minutes. Then stir in the breadcrumbs, parmesan cheese and pepper.

Butter the bottom and sides of a pie dish. Press the mushroom mix into the dish evenly on bottom and sides. Sprinkle the grated cheddar over the mixture.

In a blender (or by hand), beat the cream cheese and eggs together until well mixed. Stir in the diced ham. Then pour the mixture over the mushrooms and cheese in the pie dish. Bake for 30 minutes.

French Omelette

Chock-full of healthy ingredients, this omelette will give you the perfect start to the day.

<u>Serves 1</u>   <u>Prep time 5m</u>   <u>Cook time 10m</u>

1 mushroom
1 onion
1 clove garlic, minced
2 eggs
1 tsp basil
1 tbsp olive oil
1oz mozzarella cheese
1 tomato, chopped

Put the eggs and the basil in a bowl and whisk to a frothy consistency. Put to one side.

Then put the mushrooms, onion and garlic in a frying pan and fry them in the olive oil until cooked.

Add the egg and basil mixture to the frying pan over a medium heat and cook the omelette until it has set.

Sprinkle the mozzarella cheese over it, add the chopped tomato and serve.

Baked Eggs With Spinach

A hearty one-pot meal with a delicious combination of flavours. For a meatier dish, add chunks of cooked chicken, ham or bacon when you add the eggs.

Serves 2   **Prep time 10m**   **Cook time 40m**

200g new potatoes, thickly sliced
1 small onion, finely chopped
1 garlic clove, finely chopped
1/2 pepper, de-seeded and cut into small pieces
200g cannellini beans
2 medium tomatoes, chopped
150ml passata
1-2 tbsp Worcestershire sauce
50g spinach
2 eggs
1 handful of oregano

Boil the potatoes in a pan until they are tender and then drain them. Next, fry the onion, garlic and pepper in a frying pan for 5 minutes until they are soft.

Add them all to a large pan together with the beans, tomatoes, passata and Worcestershire sauce. Season and simmer for 10-12 minutes. Stir in the spinach. Then make four small holes in the mixture and crack an egg into each one. Cover and cook for 5 minutes. Serve garnished with the oregano.

Power Porridge

Start your day with slow-release carbohydrates and plenty of fibre with this simple porridge.

Serves 1   **Prep time 5m**   **Cook time 5m**

75g quinoa
250ml water
250ml milk
2 apples, chopped finely or grated
1/2 tsp cinnamon
1 tsp vanilla extract
1 tbsp sunflower seeds
1 tbsp almonds, ground

Rinse the quinoa under cold running water and then mix it with the water in a pan. Bring to the boil and then reduce the heat. Cover and cook for 10 minutes until the quinoa is soft.

Add the milk, chopped apple, sunflower seeds, ground almonds, cinnamon and vanilla. Cook the porridge for 5 minutes until creamy. If necessary, add more milk for a creamier texture.

Ladle into a bowl and serve.

Cinnamon Granola Bars

These granola bars are great for lunch boxes, breakfast on the run or just with a cup of coffee.

<u>Makes 10</u>   <u>Prep time 15m</u>   <u>Cook time 30m</u>

100g butter
200g porridge oats
100g sunflower seeds
50g sesame seeds
50g walnuts, chopped
1 tsp honey
1 tsp cinnamon
100g mixed berries

Heat the oven to 160°C. Butter and line the base of a medium size baking tin. Mix the oats, seeds and walnuts in a roasting tin and then put them in the oven for 5-10 minutes to toast.

Next, melt the butter and honey in a pan. Add the oat mix, cinnamon and mixed berries, then mix until the oats are well coated.

Tip into the baking tin, compact the mixture lightly and then bake it for 30 minutes.

Allow to cool in the tin before cutting into 10 bars.

Egg and Leek Bake

This hearty country dish from the Provence region of France is an easy mix of seasonal vegetables, garlic and olive oil.

Serves 2   **Prep time 5m**   **Cook time 20m**

2 eggs
1 tsp olive oil
1/2 leek, thinly sliced
100g mushrooms, sliced
1 tbsp yogurt
Pinch of black pepper

Set the oven to 170°C. Put the oil in a frying pan and add the leeks and mushrooms. Stirring regularly, cook for 5 minutes.

Then mix in the yogurt and black pepper. When done, place the mixture in an oven-proof dish and bake for 15 minutes.

Remove from the oven and serve.

Egg Ratatouille

A simple and tasty breakfast that will fuel the whole family during the day to come.

<u>Serves 2</u>   <u>Prep time 10m</u>   <u>Cook time 50m</u>

2 eggs
1 pepper, de-seeded and thinly sliced
1 courgette, diced
1 tomato
1 onion, chopped
1 garlic clove, finely chopped
1 tbsp thyme
1 tbsp olive oil

Heat the oil in a large frying pan. Put the onion, pepper, garlic, courgette and thyme in the pan and fry for 3 minutes, stirring frequently.

Next, add the tomato and 200ml of water to the pan. Bring it to the boil, cover, and then simmer for 40 minutes.

Remove the ratatouille from the heat and make two spaces in it. Crack one egg into each space. Put it back on to a medium heat and let it cook for 5 minutes.

Then serve.

Bircher Muesli

Bircher Muesli was first made over a century ago by the Swiss doctor Maximilian Bircher-Benner in his Zurich clinic. It is traditionally left overnight to soften the oats.

Serves 1   **Prep time 5m**   **Cook time 60m**

25g rolled oats
1 tsp honey
100ml semi-skimmed milk
1 apple, unpeeled and grated
1 tbsp low-fat yogurt
10g walnuts, chopped
5 raspberries

Add the honey to the oats and then place into a pan with the milk. Leave to soak until all the milk has been absorbed (this should take about one hour), or overnight in the fridge.

Then mix the grated apple into the oats, and finish by putting the yogurt, raspberries and walnuts on top.

Scrambled Eggs

The key to making scrambled eggs is whisking the eggs thoroughly before cooking them. This incorporates air, which makes them lighter and fluffier.

<u>Serves 1</u>   <u>Prep time 5m</u>   <u>Cook time 5m</u>

3 eggs
1 mushroom
1 tomato
2 slices of ham
50ml milk
2 tsp butter

Place the eggs and milk in a bowl and whisk to a smooth consistency. Chop the tomato, mushroom and ham as finely as you can and stir them into the egg mixture.

Melt the butter in a frying pan and then add the egg mixture. With the pan on a medium heat, slowly cook it while stirring continuously.

Be careful not to overcook. The heat in the pan will continue to cook and firm up the eggs after they have been removed from heat.

When the scrambled egg is firm, it is ready to eat.

Kedgeree

This version of the breakfast classic is made with salmon instead of haddock, which is high in salt; and cauliflower instead of rice, which is high in carbohydrates.

<u>Serves 2</u>   <u>Prep time 10m</u>   <u>Cook time 30m</u>

1/2 cauliflower, grated
2 eggs
2 tsp olive oil
1 onion, finely chopped
150ml semi-skimmed milk
150g salmon
1 lemon, juice of
1 tbsp low-fat yogurt
2 tbsp cumin, finely chopped

Hard boil the eggs for twelve minutes or so, shell and cut them into quarters. Put the grated cauliflower into a pan together with the milk and simmer for 5 minutes. Drain and put to one side.

Heat the olive oil in a frying pan and fry the onion for 5 minutes. Add the salmon and cook for another 5 minutes. Then add the lemon juice, yoghurt and cumin and mix thoroughly.

Finally, combine the cauliflower with the salmon/vegetable mixture and top with the quartered eggs.

Full English Breakfast

An absolute classic, the English Breakfast has been maligned for years now due to it's fat content. However, it's now thought that the same fat may actually boost the metabolism for the rest of the day, and prime the body to burn fat more efficiently.

<u>Serves 1</u>　　　　<u>Prep time 5m</u>　　　　<u>Cook time 15m</u>

2 eggs
2 slices of bacon
2 sausages
1 large mushroom, sliced
2 slices of black pudding
1 tomato, cut in two
1 tsp of olive oil

Put the olive oil in a frying pan and fry the bacon, sausages and mushroom. When done, remove and place on a side dish. Next, fry the black pudding. Remove and place on the side dish. Do the same with the tomato.

Finally, fry the two eggs. Add to the side dish and, if necessary, give it a quick blast in the microwave to get it all nice and hot.

Almond Granola

This homemade granola is a healthier version of the shop-bought varieties, which are almost always much higher in sugar.

Serves 10   **Prep time 10m**   **Cook time 25m**

250g oats
40g flaked almonds
1 egg
2 tsp of honey
50g raisins
100g apricots, chopped
1 tsp olive oil

Preheat the oven to 150°C. Place the oats and almonds in a bowl and mix. In a separate bowl, beat the egg together with the honey until a frothy consistency has been achieved. Then add the oats and almonds and combine thoroughly.

Grease a baking sheet with the olive oil. Spread the mixture onto the baking sheet, place it in the oven and bake for about 15 minutes. Finally, add the raisins and apricots and bake for 10 more minutes.

Low-Fat English Breakfast

In spite of the fact that the full English Breakfast is not now thought to be bad for you, there are still plenty of people who aren't so sure. This version is for them.

<u>Serves 1</u>   <u>Prep time 5m</u>   <u>Cook time 15m</u>

2 low-fat pork sausages
2 rashers of lean bacon, visible fat removed
1 large mushroom, quartered or sliced
1 small onion, cut into rings
1 tomato, halved
1 medium boiled potato, cubed
½ tin of baked beans
2 eggs

Grill the sausages for 5 minutes, turning frequently. Put them to one side when they are done and then grill the bacon.

Place the mushroom, onion, tomato and potato in a frying pan and fry until the mushroom, tomato and onion are softened and the potato is golden brown. Heat the beans in a small pan until ready.

Crack the eggs into a non-stick pan and cook to your liking. Assemble your breakfast on a large plate, adding brown sauce or tomato ketchup if desired.

Mushroom & Garlic Omelette

Omelettes make a fast and very filling meal, especially when they are served with salad.

<u>Serves 1</u> <u>Prep time 5m</u> <u>Cook time 10m</u>

3 eggs
100g mushrooms
1 tbsp olive oil
2 cloves garlic
1 tsp of mixed herbs
2 tbsp milk

Dice the mushrooms and garlic cloves as finely as you can. Then place in a mixing bowl with the rest of the ingredients and whisk to a frothy consistency.

Heat the olive oil in a small non-stick frying pan until it begins to bubble. Turn the heat down and then pour the mixture into the pan.

Cook the omelette until it is golden brown on the underside. Turn it over and cook for another thirty seconds or so.

Apple and Linseed Porridge

Start the day the right way with a nutrient-packed oaty breakfast - full of stomach-friendly fibre that is great for digestion.

<u>Serves 1</u>   <u>Prep time 5m</u>   <u>Cook time 6m</u>

50g rolled oats
1 apple
1 tsp ground nutmeg
250ml semi-skimmed milk
1 tbsp ground linseed
1 tsp honey

The first step is to peel and grate the apple. Then mix the grated apple with the nutmeg, oats and milk in a saucepan.

Bring to the boil then reduce the heat and cook for 5 minutes. Then stir in the ground linseed.

Pour into a breakfast bowl, add a drizzle of honey on top and your porridge is ready to eat.

Lunch Recipes

Carrot Kugel

Kugel is a traditional Jewish dish. It's usually made with noodles and is sweet, but savoury versions can be made with potatoes or carrots. It makes an excellent light lunch or supper when served with salad, and can be eaten hot or cold.

<u>Serves 2</u>   <u>Prep time 10m</u>   <u>Cook time 25m</u>

1 egg
250g carrots
25g onion, grated
25g cheddar cheese, finely grated
25g cream cheese
1 clove garlic, crushed
1 tsp mustard
1 tsp sunflower oil

Put the egg, garlic, mustard, cream cheese and cheddar cheese in a bowl and mix well.

Grate the carrots and onion, add to the egg and cheese mixture, and beat vigorously until all the ingredients are thoroughly mixed.

Oil an oven-proof pie dish or tin. Then add the Kugel mixture and lightly press to ensure it's evenly spread in the tin. Bake in an oven preheated to 180°C for 20-25 minutes and then serve.

Chicken Burritos

These burritos are quick to prepare, filling and make a substantial lunch.

<u>Serves 2</u>   <u>Prep time 15m</u>   <u>Cook time 15m</u>

80g rice
2 tsp olive oil
1 onion
1 chicken breast, cut into chunks
1 pepper, de-seeded and chopped
1 clove garlic
1 tsp chilli powder
2 tortillas
1 tbsp cream cheese

First, put the rice on to cook in a pan.

In a separate pan, fry the onion, chicken and pepper in the olive oil for about 10 minutes.

Add the chilli powder and garlic and cook for another 2 minutes or so. When the rice is cooked, add it to the chicken and onion, and mix well.

Warm the tortillas and spread a layer of cream cheese on each one. Then add the chicken and rice mixture and roll up the tortillas, tucking in the ends, to form a neat parcel.

Thai Cauliflower Rice

This low calorie meal is perfect for a quick lunch. Rather than use carbohydrate-high rice though, the recipe uses grated cauliflower as a healthier substitute.

<u>Serves 2</u>   <u>Prep time 10m</u>   <u>Cook time 10m</u>

2 tsp olive oil
1 onion
1/2 pepper, de-seeded and chopped
70g pineapple, cut into small chunks
2 tbsp Thai green curry paste
1/2 cauliflower, grated
70g peas
100g can bamboo shoots, drained
100g prawns
150ml semi-skimmed milk

Heat the olive oil in a frying pan and fry the onion for 2 minutes. Stir in the pepper, pineapple and the green curry paste and cook for 3 more minutes.

Put the cauliflower in a pan with the milk and simmer it for five minutes. Then drain the milk and return the cauliflower to the pan.

Stir the peas, bamboo shoots and prawns into the 'cauliflower rice', then cook for 2 or 3 minutes until the prawns are hot and the peas tender. Then add the onion and pepper mixture, stir well and serve.

Duck Stir Fry

Duck meat is lean and full of flavour, unlike much of the chicken sold these days. This meal goes well with rice.

<u>Serves 2</u>   <u>Prep time 10m</u>   <u>Cook time 15m</u>

4 duck breasts
1 tsp Chinese Five Spice
300g pak choi (Chinese cabbage)
2 tbsp olive oil
2 peppers, de-seeded and sliced
150g sugar snap peas, sliced lengthways
3cm root ginger, finely chopped
1 red chilli, de-seeded and sliced
100g black bean sauce
1 tsp coriander

Roughly chop the pak choi – keep the stalk and leaf ends separate.

Heat half the oil in a frying pan and stir-fry the duck for five minutes. Put into a bowl and set aside. Heat the remaining oil and fry the peppers, sugar snap peas and pak choi stalks for a few minutes until they are soft. Add the ginger, pak choi leaves, chilli and the five spice powder and fry for a couple more minutes.

Return the duck to the pan together with the black bean sauce and 100ml of water. Heat through, sprinkle with the coriander and serve.

Salmon & Avocado Burger

A variation on the standard hamburger, the Salmon & Avocado Burger is not just healthier, it is considerably tastier.

<u>Serves 2</u>   <u>Prep time 5m</u>   <u>Cook time 10m</u>

2 spring onions, roughly chopped
1 handful of parsley
1 handful of rocket
250g salmon fillets
1/2 avocado, sliced
50g fresh breadcrumbs
1 tsp hot horseradish sauce
1 egg
1 tbsp olive oil

Using a food processor, mix the spring onions, parsley, avocado and salmon until finely chopped. Put the mixture into a large bowl and stir in the breadcrumbs, horseradish sauce, the egg and some seasoning.

Shape the mixture into 4 patties. Heat the olive oil in a large non-stick frying pan over a low-medium heat and then fry the patties for 5 minutes on either side, or until golden and cooked through.

Serve the burgers on a bed of rocket and a wedge of lemon or lime.

Mushroom Penne

Add protein to a vegan pasta dish by using a low-fat hummus in the sauce. With the mushrooms and low-carb pasta, you have a healthy and filling lunch.

Serves 2   **Prep time 20m**   **Cook time 15m**

200g chickpeas
1 tbsp lemon juice
1 garlic clove
1 tsp vegetable bouillon
2 tsp tahini
¼ tsp ground coriander
115g low-carb penne pasta
2 tsp olive oil
2 onions, halved and sliced
200g mushrooms, roughly chopped
1 handful of parsley

The first step is to put the pasta on to cook. Then make the hummus. Do this by tipping the chickpeas into a bowl with the lemon juice, garlic, bouillon, tahini and coriander. With a blender, mix to a wet paste.

Heat the oil in a pan and fry the onions and mushrooms. Drain the pasta and tip in the onion and mushroom mix. Remove from the heat and mix in the houmous and parsley. Squeeze the lemon juice over and serve.

Poached Plaice

Fillets of poached plaice in fish stock, served on a bed of samphire, make a light and succulent lunch.

<u>Serves 2</u>   <u>Prep time 10m</u>   <u>Cook time 20m</u>

150g carrots, halved lengthways
6 spring onions, chopped
400g samphire
5g dill, roughly chopped, plus 4 sprigs to serve
1 vegetable stock cube, dissolved in 500ml water
2 plaice fillets
1 tsp cornflour, dissolved in 1 tbsp skimmed milk
1 tbsp Greek yogurt

Cook the carrots in a pan of water.

Put the spring onions, dill and samphire in a pan with the plaice on top. Pour in the vegetable stock and bring to the boil. Cover and simmer for 5 minutes.

When the fish is cooked, remove it from the pan. Then put the carrots, spring onions and samphire onto plates and place the fish on top.

Stir the cornflour into the boiling stock until thickened, then add the yogurt. Mix well, then pour over the fish. Sprinkle with pepper and serve with a wedge of lemon and a sprig of dill.

Spicy Avocado Wraps

A tasty, healthy, and extremely quick and easy meal to prepare.

<u>Serves 2</u>   <u>Prep time 5m</u>   <u>Cook time 8m</u>

150g of Quorn chicken-style pieces
1 avocado
1 pepper, de-seeded and chopped
½ tsp chilli powder
1 garlic clove, chopped
1 tbsp olive oil
2 tortilla wraps
1 handful of coriander, chopped
1 lime, juice of

Mix the chicken-style pieces with the lime juice, chilli powder and garlic. Then pile it all into a frying pan and fry in the olive oil for 2 or 3 minutes.

Add the chopped pepper and fry until the pepper is cooked.

Squash half the avocado meat on to each tortilla wrap and then add the chicken-style piece mix. Sprinkle the coriander over it all, roll up the tortilla wraps and you're ready to eat.

Ginger Garlic Salmon

Another extremely quick and easy lunch to prepare. I do, however, advise you not to eat salmon bought in supermarkets or labelled as 'Atlantic salmon'. They all come from fish farms and are exposed to pollutants such as dioxin and DDT, not to mention carcinogens. These chemicals can cause a range of health issues.

Alaskan salmon is what you want - it is actually illegal to farm Alaskan salmon.

<u>Serves 2</u>   <u>Prep time 5m</u>   <u>Cook time 10m</u>

2 salmon fillets
75g butter
1 tbsp soy sauce
1 clove garlic
3cm root ginger, finely chopped or grated
1 tsp brown sugar
1 lemon, juice of

Preheat the oven grill. Then grill the salmon for about five minutes on both sides.

Heat the butter in a small saucepan and then add the soy sauce, garlic, ginger, brown sugar and lemon juice. Cook until nice and hot.

When done, pour the ginger garlic butter over the cooked salmon and serve.

Lentil Curry

This tasty vegetarian curry is perfect for a quick and easy supper.

<u>Serves 4</u>   <u>Prep time 10m</u>   <u>Cook time 25m</u>

3 tbsp olive oil
1 onion, finely chopped
1 garlic clove, finely chopped
2cm root ginger, grated
2 tsp ground coriander
2 tsp ground cumin
1/2 tsp ground turmeric
75g red or yellow lentils
150ml vegetable stock
1 cauliflower, cut into small florets
1 large carrot, diced
400ml can coconut milk
75g green beans
1 tbsp lemon juice
Salt and pepper
1 sprig of fresh coriander

Heat 2 tablespoons of the olive oil in a large saucepan and gently cook the onion for 10 minutes, stirring frequently, until soft. Add the garlic, ginger, coriander, cumin and turmeric and cook for 2 more minutes, stirring continuously.

Cont'd

Stir in the lentils, then pour in the vegetable stock. Bring to the boil, then reduce the heat, cover and gently simmer for 10 minutes.

Meanwhile, heat the remaining olive oil in a frying pan and fry the cauliflower for 2–3 minutes until lightly browned. Then add it to the lentil mixture together with the carrot and coconut milk.

Bring the curry back to a gentle simmer and cook for a further 10 minutes or until the vegetables are tender. Stir in the beans and cook for 3–4 minutes.

Add the chopped coriander and lemon juice then season to taste with salt and pepper. Transfer the curry to a warmed serving dish and garnish it with a sprig of fresh coriander.

Oriental Steamed Fish

Steaming keeps in all the goodness and flavour, while the oriental flavours of chilli, ginger and lemon work brilliantly with white fish.

<u>Serves 2</u>   <u>Prep time 10m</u>   <u>Cook time 15m</u>

2 fish fillets
2cm root ginger, chopped
1 garlic clove, chopped
1 red chilli, finely chopped
1 lime, grated zest of
1 tbsp lime juice
1 pak choi, chopped
2 tbsp soy sauce

Place the fish fillets side by side on a large square of foil and then sprinkle the ginger, garlic, chilli and lime zest over them.

Drizzle the lime juice on top and then sprinkle the pieces of pak choi around and on top of the fish. Pour the soy sauce over everything and loosely seal the foil to make a package - make sure you leave space at the top for the steam to circulate as the fish cooks.

Steam for 15 minutes. If you haven't got a steamer, put the package on a heatproof plate over a pan of gently simmering water, cover with a lid and steam.

Thai Chilli Satay

This recipe uses Shirataki noodles, which are also known as 'miracle noodles', due to their very low carbohydrate content.

Serves 4   **Prep time 5m**   **Cook time 10m**

3 tbsp crunchy peanut butter
3 tbsp sweet chilli sauce
2 tbsp soy sauce
300g Shirataki noodles
1 tbsp olive oil
2cm root ginger, grated
300g pack mixed stir-fry vegetables
1 handful of basil leaves

Mix the peanut butter, chilli sauce, 100ml water and soy sauce to make a smooth satay sauce. Put the noodles in a bowl and pour boiling water over them. Stir gently to separate, then drain thoroughly.

Heat the oil in a frying pan or wok, then stir-fry the ginger and harder pieces of veg from the stir-fry mix, such as peppers, for 2 minutes. Add the noodles and the rest of the vegetables, then stir-fry over a high heat for 1-2 minutes until the vegetables are cooked.

Add the satay sauce to the pan and mix with the vegetables and noodles. Cook until hot then put on serving plates. Sprinkle with the basil leaves to finish.

Five-Spice Pork

Chinese 5 spice powder, with it's special blend of five classic spices, garlic and pepper, adds a delicious and distinctive flavour to this pork and vegetable stir fry.

<u>Serves 2</u>   <u>Prep time 20m</u>   <u>Cook time 15m</u>

200g pork fillet, cut into strips
15g egg noodles
1 tbsp olive oil
1 small onion, finely chopped
1 garlic clove, crushed
1 tbsp five-spice powder
150g sugar snap peas
1 pepper, de-seeded and thinly sliced
50ml hot vegetable stock

Cook the noodles in boiling water for five minutes. Drain and set aside. Then stir-fry the onion and garlic in the olive oil for one minute. Put the five-spice powder in next and fry for another minute.

Add the pork strips to the pan and stir-fry for three minutes. Next in are the sugar snap peas and the pepper - stir-fry for a further 2 minutes. Pour in the stock, stir well and bring to the boil.

Add the noodles to the pan, and stir and toss until all the ingredients are well combined. Serve.

Pakistani Chickpeas

Tender cooked chickpeas are simmered lightly with tomatoes, lemon juice and onions in a spicy blend of toasted cumin seeds and chilli powder.

<u>Serves 2</u>   <u>Prep time 10m</u>   <u>Cook time 20m</u>

1 onion, chopped
1 tomato, chopped
200g chickpeas
1 tbsp olive oil
1 tsp cumin seeds
1/2 tsp salt
1/2 tsp chilli powder
1 tbsp lemon juice

Heat the cumin seeds in the olive oil until they turn a dark shade of brown.

Add the salt and chilli powder, and mix well. Stir in the chopped tomato and when the juice begins to thicken, add the chickpeas and mix well.

Finally, add the onion and lemon juice. Cook until the onion is soft. Remove from heat and serve immediately.

While it's a fact that chickpeas have quite a high level of carbohydrates, when eaten in conjunction with healthy oils and vegetables, the carbs are released slowly and so don't cause a spike in blood sugar levels.

Salmon Fish Cakes

If you're after something that's a bit lighter than potato-packed fish cakes, try this simple oriental-style version.

<u>Serves 4</u>   <u>Prep time 20m</u>   <u>Cook time 10m</u>

4 salmon fillets, cut into chunks
2 tbsp Thai red curry paste
2cm root ginger, grated
1 tsp soy sauce
1 bunch coriander, chopped
1 tsp olive oil
1 lemon, cut into wedges
2 carrots
1 small cucumber
2 tbsp white wine vinegar
1 tsp caster sugar

Put the salmon into a food processor with the curry paste, ginger, soy sauce and chopped coriander. Pulse until roughly minced. Remove the mixture and shape it into four burger-size cakes.

Heat the oil in a frying pan then fry the cakes for 4-5 minutes on each side. Next, peel strips of carrot and cucumber into a bowl. Toss with the vinegar and sugar until the sugar has dissolved, then toss through the coriander leaves. Divide the salad between four plates. Serve with the fish cakes together with the lemon.

Quinoa Pilaf

This creamy pilaf combines fluffy, nutty-flavoured quinoa with a delicious cheese to give a most unusual flavour and texture.

<u>Serves 1</u>   <u>Prep time 10m</u>   <u>Cook time 30m</u>

4 tbsp quinoa
3 tbsp olive oil
2 tbsp raw sunflower seeds
2 cloves garlic, minced
50g spinach leaves
2 tsp lemon juice
25g grated hard cheese, such as cheddar

Bring a pot of lightly salted water to the boil. Add the quinoa and cook until it is soft. Drain and set aside.

Heat the olive oil in a frying pan, stir in the sunflower seeds and cook for about 2 minutes until lightly toasted. Stir in the garlic and cook for 2 more minutes.

Add the cooled quinoa and spinach leaves and stir until the quinoa is hot and the spinach has wilted.

Add the lemon juice and all but a pinch of the cheese. Stir until the cheese has melted. Serve sprinkled with the remaining cheese.

Dinner Recipes

Jollof Chicken Rice

A popular West African dish that's cooked in one pan and is ideal for a simple, quick and tasty dinner.

<u>Serves 4</u>   <u>Prep time 15m</u>   <u>Cook time 30m</u>

2 tsp olive oil
1 large onion, chopped
350g chicken breast, cut into chunks
1 red pepper, chopped
1 yellow pepper, chopped
400g dry Shirataki rice
2 garlic cloves, crushed
3 cm ginger, finely chopped
1 Scotch Bonnet chilli, chopped
2 tbsp tomato purée
1 chicken stock cube dissolved in 450ml water
400g can chopped tomatoes
100g okra, chopped into 2cm pieces
2 tbsp chopped coriander

Heat the oil in a large pan then add the onion and cook for 3-4 minutes until it's starting to brown.

Add the chicken chunks and cook for a further 3-4 minutes, stirring regularly to make sure the chicken cooks evenly.

Next into the pan is the red and yellow peppers. Carry

Cont'd

on cooking for another 2 minutes before adding the garlic, ginger, chilli and tomato puree. Mix thoroughly and then add the rice, chicken stock and tomatoes. Bring to the boil, reduce the heat, cover and simmer for 10 minutes or so.

Scatter the okra on top of the rice, replace the lid and simmer a further 5 minutes.

Now turn off the heat but don't remove the lid. Leave to stand for 5 minutes. Add the coriander, give it one last stir and serve.

Note: Shirataki rice and noodles are both made from the root of a plant called Konnyaku. As they are made from the soluble fibre of the plant, they are extremely low in calories.

Prawn Biryani

A fragrantly spiced pilaf-style dish that doesn't take much more effort than ringing for a take-away yet is far healthier. Grated cauliflower is used instead of rice.

<u>Serves 4</u>   <u>Prep time 15m</u>   <u>Cook time 15m</u>

400g can chopped tomatoes
300g baby leaf spinach, chopped
2 tbsp olive oil
1 onion, thinly sliced
1 red chilli, de-seeded and thinly sliced
1cm root ginger, finely chopped
1 tbsp ground cumin
1 tbsp ground coriander
1 tsp ground turmeric
½ tsp ground nutmeg
1/2 cauliflower, grated
1 pinch of sugar
225g peeled tiger prawns

Sieve the tomatoes over a heatproof measuring jug, place in a bowl and then set aside. Keep the sieved juice that's in the jug. Put a kettle of water on to boil.

Heat the oil in a large flame-proof casserole dish over a medium heat. Add the onion, chilli and ginger, and stir for 3 minutes.

Cont'd

Stir in the cumin, coriander, turmeric and nutmeg and continue stirring until the onion is cooked. Add the grated cauliflower and drained tomatoes to the casserole and stir to mix with the spices.

Add enough boiling water to the reserved tomato juice to make up to 450ml. Stir this liquid and the sugar into the casserole, add a pinch of salt, then bring to the boil.

Reduce the heat to low, cover tightly and leave the 'cauliflower rice' to cook without lifting the lid for 10–12 minutes.

Then stir in the spinach in small batches, adding more as each addition wilts. When all the spinach has been added, lay the prawns on top, re-cover the casserole and turn the heat down to very low.

Cook for 2 minutes, then turn off the heat and leave to stand for 1 minute, without lifting the lid. By this time the spinach will have wilted further and the prawns will have cooked through. Gently fork together to combine the cauliflower rice, spinach and prawns and then serve immediately.

Chicken & Chorizo Jambalaya

A Cajun-inspired rice pot recipe with spicy Spanish sausage, sweet peppers and tomatoes. Low-carb dry Shirataki rice is used instead of normal rice.

<u>Serves 4</u>   <u>Prep time 10m</u>   <u>Cook time 35m</u>

2 chicken breasts, chopped
1 onion, chopped
1 red pepper, thinly sliced
250g dry Shirataki rice
400g can plum tomatoes
2 garlic cloves, crushed
1 tbsp olive oil
75g chorizo, sliced
1 tbsp Cajun seasoning
350ml chicken stock

Heat the oil in a large frying pan and cook the chicken for 5 minutes or so. Remove and set aside.

Add the onion and cook for 3-4 minutes until soft. Then add the pepper, garlic, chorizo and Cajun seasoning, and cook for another 5 minutes.

Cook the Shirataki rice by simmering it in a separate pan of water for 20 minutes. Then drain the water and add the rice, the chicken and the chicken stock to the pan containing the pepper, garlic, chorizo and Cajun seasoning. Mix well and serve.

Sausage Stew

Sausages are a favourite food all over the world. This recipe presents them in a somewhat unusual way.

Serves 4   **Prep time 10m**   **Cook time 20m**

8 sausages
1 tsp olive oil
2 tsp dried oregano
2 garlic cloves, sliced
400g can chopped tomatoes
200ml beef stock
100g pitted black olives in brine
500g mushrooms, thickly sliced

Cut the sausages into meatball-size pieces. Then heat a large pan and fry the sausage pieces in the oil for about 5 minutes until browned all over.

Add the oregano and garlic, fry for 1 more minute, then add the tomatoes, stock, olives and mushrooms.

Simmer for 15 minutes until the sausages are cooked through and the sauce has thickened. Serve the sausage stew with mashed potato or pasta.

Venison Stir-Fry

Venison is a lovely, tasty meat. It also has half the calories and just one sixth of the amount of saturated fat found in beef. Give it a try with this delicious stir-fry.

<u>Serves 2</u>   **<u>Prep time 15m</u>**   **<u>Cook time 10m</u>**

2 tbsp sesame oil
8 cherry tomatoes
300g venison, cut into thin strips
1 small leek, cut into fine strips
1/2 pepper, finely sliced
1 tbsp soy sauce
3 tbsp sweet chilli dipping sauce
3 tbsp olive oil
Salt and pepper

Heat 1 tbsp of sesame oil in a pan and fry the tomatoes for two minutes. Add the venison, leek and pepper, and stir-fry for a further 5 minutes. Then add the soy sauce and cook for another 3 minutes. Season with salt and pepper to taste.

To make the dressing, mix the sweet chilli sauce, olive oil and 1 tbsp of sesame oil together in a small bowl.

To serve, place the venison stir fry on a serving platter and drizzle with the dressing.

Tandoori Chicken

This low-fat curried chicken is packed full of flavour. It's quick to cook and the marinade does all the work.

<u>Serves 4</u>   <u>Prep time 30m</u>   <u>Cook time 15m</u>

8 chicken thighs
1 red onion, finely chopped
1 lemon, juice of
2 tsp paprika
1 tsp olive oil

For the marinade:
300ml Greek yogurt
2cm root ginger, grated
2 garlic cloves, crushed
1/2 tsp garam masala
1/2 tsp ground cumin
¼ tsp turmeric

Mix the lemon juice with the paprika and red onion in a large shallow dish. Slash the chicken thighs then turn them in the juice and put to one side.

Mix the marinade and pour over the chicken. Cover and chill for at least one hour.

Place the chicken pieces onto a hot grill. Brush with a little olive oil and grill until lightly charred and completely cooked through. Serve.

Creamy Courgette Lasagne

Quick, easy to prepare and meat-free, this lasagne is ideal for vegetarians.

Serves 4   **Prep time 10m**   **Cook time 20m**

9 low-carb lasagne sheets
1 tbsp olive oil
1 onion, finely chopped
3 courgettes, finely chopped
2 garlic cloves, crushed
250g tub ricotta
50g cheddar cheese, grated
350g jar pasta tomato sauce

Pre-heat the oven to 220°C. Cook the lasagne sheets for about 5 minutes until soft. Rinse and then drizzle with a little oil to stop them sticking together.

In a frying pan, fry the onion in the olive oil. After 3 minutes, add the chopped courgette and garlic and keep frying until the courgette has softened. Stir in two thirds of both the ricotta and the cheddar cheese, then season to taste. Heat the tomato sauce until hot.

In a large baking dish, layer the ingredients starting with half the courgette mix, then pasta, then tomato sauce. Repeat, top with blobs of the remaining ricotta, then scatter the rest of the cheddar. Bake in the oven for about 10 minutes before serving.

Spicy Chicken & Broccoli Stir Fry

Garlic, dried red chillies and chilli paste add some spice to chicken and broccoli.

Serves 4   **Prep time 20m**   **Cook time 30m**

275g broccoli florets
1 tbsp olive oil
2 chicken breast fillets cut into strips
1/2 bunch spring onions, sliced
4 cloves garlic, thinly sliced
1 tbsp hoisin sauce
1 tbsp chilli paste
1 tbsp light soy sauce
1/2 tsp ground ginger
1/4 tsp dried crushed chillies
4 tbsp chicken stock

Cook the broccoli in a steamer until it's tender but still firm. Heat the oil in a frying pan over a medium heat and stir-fry the chicken, spring onions and garlic until the chicken is cooked.

Add the hoisin sauce, chilli paste and soy sauce to the frying pan. Season with the ginger, chillies, salt and black pepper. Then stir in the chicken stock and simmer for about 2 minutes.

Finally, mix in the steamed broccoli until it's well coated with the sauce mixture. Serve.

Pepper Ciambotta

Ciambotta is a vegetable stew, the ingredients of which can vary according to what's on hand. It makes a delicious accompaniment to roasted chicken, fish or meat.

<u>Serves 4</u>　　　<u>Prep time 15m</u>　　　<u>Cook time 45m</u>

2 tbsp olive oil
1 large onion, chopped
2 small fennel bulbs
2 cloves of garlic
1 pepper, chopped
1 can tomatoes
2 medium courgettes, chopped
200g green beans, chopped
1 handful of basil leaves

Heat the olive oil and then add the onion and fennel. Cook for 15 minutes or until the vegetables are lightly browned and tender, stirring occasionally. Add the pepper and garlic, and cook for another 5-7 minutes.

Add the tomatoes with their juice, the courgettes, green beans and 1/2 teaspoon of salt. Raise the heat to medium-high, stirring and breaking up the tomatoes. Then lower the heat to medium-low, cover, and simmer for 2530 minutes or until all the vegetables are tender. Top with the basil and serve.

Barbecue Pork Steaks

Pork steaks marinated in garlic and lemon, cooked with apple and red onion. These can be barbecued, cooked in a griddle pan or grilled.

<u>Serves 4</u>   <u>Prep time 20m</u>   <u>Cook time 15m</u>

4 lean pork loin steaks
6 cloves garlic, crushed
1 lemon, juice of
2 apples
2 red onions
2 tsp balsamic vinegar

Put the pork, garlic and lemon juice in a food bag, seal it and then give it a good shake so the pork is thoroughly coated. Put it to one side. De-core the apples and cut them into 16 wedges. Slice the onions into rings leaving the skin on - this holds them together.

Put the apple wedges and slices of onion onto the BBQ, or griddle pan, and grill for about 10 minutes turning as necessary. When the onions are cooked, remove their skin and drizzle the vinegar onto them.

Cook the pork steaks for 3-5 minutes on each side, depending on thickness. When done, remove them from the barbecue and cover with foil. Leave to rest for 3-4 minutes, before serving with the onion and apple.

Chilli Casserole

Chilli casserole can be served by itself in bowls with grated cheese and sour cream. It can also be eaten with rice.

<u>Serves 4</u>   <u>Prep time 5m</u>   <u>Cook time 20m</u>

1 onion, sliced
500g mince meat
2 cloves garlic, crushed
1 pepper, diced
200g can tomatoes
2 tsp tomato paste
100g grated cheese
2 tsp ground cumin
2 tsp ground coriander
1 tsp chilli powder

Fry the onion and garlic until soft, add the mince and cook until all the meat has browned. Add the pepper and cook until it's soft.

Add all the other ingredients, stir and cook for about 5 minutes. Then pour into a baking dish. Sprinkle the grated cheese on top and cook at 180°C for 20 minutes.

Garnish with sour cream and a sprinkle of coriander, divide into four bowls and then serve.

Almond Nachos

Nachos are a very popular Mexican dish, an important ingredient of which is tortilla chips. Made with almond flour, the chips in this recipe are low-carb and very good for you.

<u>Serves 6</u>   <u>Prep time 20m</u>   <u>Cook time 20m</u>

Tortilla Chips
170g mozzarella cheese, grated
85g almond flour
2 tbsp cream cheese
1 egg
1 tsp cumin
1 tsp coriander
1 tsp chilli powder
2 tsp olive oil

Nacho Meat Sauce
1 onion, diced
500g minced meat
400g can tomatoes, chopped
1 tbsp tomato paste

To make the meat sauce, fry the diced onion in the olive oil and then add and cook the minced meat for about 5 minutes. Add the tomatoes and tomato paste. Stir, then leave it to simmer over a low heat for 15 minutes whilst

Cont'd

you make the tortilla chips and toppings.

To make the tortilla chips, mix the grated cheese and almond flour in a bowl. Then add the cream cheese and microwave on HIGH for one minute.

Stir then microwave on HIGH for another 30 seconds. Remove and stir again. Add the egg and the spices. Mix thoroughly to a pastry-like consistency.

Place the 'pastry' between 2 sheets of baking paper and roll it into a thin rectangle. Remove the top piece of baking paper and slide the baking paper with the pastry onto a baking tray and bake at 220C for 12-15 minutes, or until brown on the top. Flip the pastry over and brown the other side.

Once cooked, remove the pastry from the oven and cut it into tortilla chip triangle shapes. Bake again at 220°C for 3-5 minutes.

To put it all together, place a handful of the tortilla chips on a plate. Ladle the meat sauce over the chips and then add the grated cheese, which will melt on the hot meat sauce. Serve with a side salad if desired.

Vegetable Paella

Perfect for vegetarians, but great for meat-eaters too, this hearty rice dish made with low-carb dry Shirataki rice is wonderfully rich and satisfying.

<u>Serves 4</u>   <u>Prep time 15m</u>   <u>Cook time 30m</u>

3 tbsp olive oil
1 onion, chopped
2 garlic cloves, crushed
2 courgettes, chopped
2 carrots, peeled and chopped
250g dry Shirataki rice
200g chopped tomatoes
1 tsp turmeric
1 tsp paprika
800ml vegetable stock
100g French beans, chopped
100g frozen peas
2 tbsp parsley, chopped

Heat the oil in a frying pan. Add the onion and garlic, and cook for 2 minutes without letting them brown. Add the courgettes, carrots and vegetable stock. Cook for another 5 minutes or so over a high heat, stirring constantly. When done, put to one side.

Next, cook the Shirataki rice by simmering it in water for 20 minutes. Drain the water.

Cont'd

When the rice is ready, add it to the pan that contains the vegetables. Give it all a good stir and then add the tomatoes with their juice, and the turmeric and paprika.

Now cook the beans and peas in boiling water for 5 minutes. Drain and add both to the rice and vegetables.

Cook for a couple of minutes to make sure everything is good and hot, sprinkle the parsley on top and then serve.

Chinese Braised Beef

The perfect dinner when you fancy something hearty and warming. It comes with some exotic flavours as well that are sure to intrigue you.

<u>Serves 4</u>   <u>Prep time 10m</u>   <u>Cook time 120m</u>

2 tbsp olive oil
1 glass red wine
3 cloves of garlic, thinly sliced
3cm piece of root ginger, grated
1 bunch of spring onions, sliced
1 red chilli, de-seeded and sliced
1½ kg braising beef, cut into large chunks
2 tbsp plain flour
1 tsp Chinese five-spice powder
2 tbsp dark soy sauce
300ml beef stock

Heat the olive oil in a large frying pan and fry the garlic, ginger, onions and chilli for 3 minutes until soft. Put on a plate and place to one side.

Toss the beef in the flour then put it in the frying pan in batches as necessary. Cook each batch for about 5 minutes until brown.

Add the five-spice powder to the pan together with the

Cont'd

onion, garlic, ginger and chilli mixture and fry it for 2 minutes or so. Lastly, splash in the wine.

Transfer everything to a casserole dish and add the soy sauce and beef stock.

Place the cover on the casserole dish and put it in an oven pre-heated to 150°C .

Cook for 2 hours stirring the meat halfway through. The meat should be very soft, and any sinewy bits should have melted. It will now be ready to eat.

Basmati rice is the perfect complement to Chinese braised beef.

Chicken And Leek Pie

Low in carbohydrates thanks to the almond flour, this chicken and leek pie is the basis of a dinner that the whole family will enjoy.

<u>Serves 6</u>   <u>Prep time 20m</u>   <u>Cook time 30m</u>

Pie Crust
55g butter
100g almond meal flour
1/2 tsp salt
1 egg
1 tbsp psyllium husk
2 tbsp coconut flour

Pie Filling
55g butter
1 leek, chopped
800g chicken, diced
200g cream cheese
200g cheddar cheese, grated
4 eggs
Salt and pepper

To make the crust, melt the butter and then add it to a bowl together with the almond flour and salt. Mix well. Then add the egg, psyllium husk and coconut flour, and mix again until a dough is formed.

Cont'd

Press the dough into a greased and lined pie dish with deep sides, or a casserole dish. Put it in the oven and bake at 180°C for 10 minutes or until just starting to brown. Remove from the oven.

To make the pie filling, melt the butter in a pan and add the chopped leek. Cook for 5 minutes, stirring occasionally, until it's cooked.

Remove the leek from the pan and put it to one side. Using the same pan, now cook the diced chicken.

When the chicken is cooked, reduce the heat, add the cream cheese and stir until it melts. Cook gently for a further 3-5 minutes.

Now put all the pie filling ingredients into a large bowl and mix them thoroughly. Then add the eggs and mix again.

Pour the pie filling into the cooked pie crust, place it in the oven and bake at 180°C for about 20 minutes until golden on top.

Cauliflower Pizza

This dish is a sneaky way to get more veggies into your children. The cheese masks the 'cauliflower' flavour.

<u>Serves 4</u>   <u>Prep time 20m</u>   <u>Cook time 20m</u>

1 medium cauliflower, finely chopped
1 egg
100g grated mozzarella cheese
1 tbsp each of rosemary and oregano
Salt and pepper

Cut the cauliflower into small pieces, put them in a food processor and blitz until quite fine. Then steam them until they are soft, or microwave for 5 minutes. Place the cauliflower onto a clean tea towel and twist to remove all the liquid - if not enough liquid is removed, the pizza base won't crisp. Put the drained cauliflower in a large mixing bowl and add the egg, seasoning, herbs and grated cheese. Mix until a dough is formed.

Prepare a baking tray lined with a sheet of baking paper. Place the ball of 'cauliflower dough' onto the baking sheet and press it into a round pizza shape.

Brush the top with some olive oil to help it crisp, then bake at 180°C for 15 minutes or until golden. Finally, add the desired toppings, cover with more cheese and cook until the cheese is melted and bubbling. Then serve.

Beef Goulash

A fancy way of dressing up stewing beef. It's spicy but not mouth-burningly so!

Serves 6   **Prep time 20m**   **Cook time 150m**

1kg braising steak
1 tbsp olive oil
2 onions, sliced
4 garlic cloves, crushed
2 tbsp paprika
1 beef stock cube
500ml cold water
400g can chopped tomatoes
2 tbsp tomato purée
2 bay leaves
2 peppers
Salt and pepper

Preheat the oven to 170°C. Cut the meat into 5cm chunks and season with salt and pepper.

Heat the olive oil in a large flame-proof casserole dish and then add the meat and fry until it's nicely browned.

Next, put the onions in the dish and cook with the meat for 5 minutes until they are soft. Add the crushed garlic and cook for a further minute, stirring regularly.

Cont'd

Sprinkle the paprika over the meat and crumble the beef stock cube on top. Then add the water, tomatoes, tomato purée and bay leaves. Stir well and bring to a simmer. Then put the lid on the dish and transfer it to the oven. While the meat is cooking, remove the core and seeds from the peppers and cut them into small chunks.

After one and a half hours, remove the dish from the oven. Stir in the peppers, put the lid back on and place the goulash back in the oven for a further hour or until the beef is tender. Then serve.

Nut Roast

A satiating vegetarian loaf packed with nuts, fruit, spices and vegetables that is just perfect for an evening meal.

Serves 4   **Prep time 15m**   **Cook time 60m**

100g butternut squash
2 tbsp olive oil
1 onion, finely chopped
1 pepper, finely chopped
2 cloves garlic, crushed
150g mixed unsalted nuts
2 eggs
150g ground almonds
200g cooked chestnuts, finely chopped
2 tbsp water
1 tsp ground nutmeg
250g spinach
25g dried cranberries

First, cook the spinach. To do this, heat 1 tablespoon of olive oil in a pan and then start adding the spinach, a handful at a time. As each handful wilts, add another. Cook for a couple of minutes, stirring the spinach constantly. When done, put to one side.

De-seed the butternut squash and cut it into chunks. Place the chunks in a pan of boiling water and boil until

Cont'd

tender. Then mash them and put to one side.

Next, heat the remaining olive oil in a pan and add the onion, stirring regularly. When it's starting to brown, add the pepper and cook for about 5 minutes. Add the garlic, mix, remove from the heat and allow to cool.

Divide the nuts into 3 piles. Put one pile aside, roughly chop the second pile and finely chop the third pile.

Add the eggs to a bowl with the ground almonds, onion, pepper, finely chopped and roughly chopped nuts, the chestnuts, water and nutmeg. Mix thoroughly.

Rub olive oil around a 1lb loaf tin and line it with greaseproof paper. Then take two-thirds of the egg mixture and press it around the tin to line it, leaving room in the centre for the filling. Add the butternut squash followed by a layer of spinach in the centre. Sprinkle the cranberries on top. Next, add the rest of the egg mixture to create a lid and sprinkle with the reserved whole nuts, pressing them gently into the topping.

Cover with a piece of foil and place the loaf in another, larger, oven dish. Fill it with water to half way up the loaf tin. Cook in the oven for 30 minutes at 170°C, then remove the foil and cook for another 10 minutes. Remove from the oven, turn out onto a plate and serve.

Aubergine & Courgette Bake

This recipe is a much healthier version of a classic Italian dish.

<u>Serves 4</u>   <u>Prep time 30m</u>   <u>Cook time 50m</u>

2 large aubergines, cut into chunks
2 courgettes, cut into strips
1 tbsp olive oil
1 onion, finely chopped
1 red pepper, finely chopped
2 cloves garlic, crushed
400g can chopped tomatoes
50g parmesan cheese, finely grated
120g mozzarella cheese, thinly sliced

Grill the aubergines and courgettes until they are browned on each side. Next, heat the olive oil in a pan and fry the onion. Then add the red pepper, stirring constantly for 5 minutes. Mix in the garlic and tomatoes, and allow to simmer for 5 minutes.

Add some of the sauce to an oven-proof dish and put some of the aubergine and courgette slices on top. Then add more sauce and sprinkle with parmesan cheese. Repeat to create layers and top the final layer with the slices of mozzarella cheese. Place the dish in the oven and bake for 30–40 minutes at 180°C

Mushroom Risotto

A creamy risotto made with barley rather than rice and topped with a variety of mushrooms.

<u>Serves 4</u>   <u>Prep time 15m</u>   <u>Cook time 40m</u>

2 tsp olive oil
400g mixed mushrooms, sliced
1 onion, chopped
1 pepper, chopped
250g pearl barley
2 cloves of garlic, crushed
1 stock cube in 700ml boiling water
1 tbsp chopped basil
4 tbsp cream

Heat the olive oil in a pan and fry the onion. Add the pepper and garlic and cook for 2 minutes, then add the mixed mushrooms and cook for 2-3 minutes more.

Put a handful of mushrooms aside to garnish the dish.

Stir in the barley, add the stock and mix well. Bring to the boil, then turn down the heat and simmer until the liquid is absorbed. The barley should be cooked but still firm.

Stir in the cream and the basil, scatter the reserved mushrooms on top to garnish and serve.

Fish Stew

A hearty Mediterranean seafood dinner, packed with vegetables and garlic.

Serves 4   **Prep time 15m**   **Cook time 20m**

1 carrot, diced
1 fish stock cube in 600ml of water
1/2 bulb fennel, sliced
1 pepper, sliced
1 leek, chopped
1 tsp turmeric
2 cloves garlic, crushed
2 tsp olive oil
4 x fish fillets, cut in half to give 8 pieces
150g king prawns
150g mussel meat
2 tomatoes, chopped
1 tbsp finely chopped parsley

Put the water in a pan with the stock cube, bring to the boil, then turn down the heat. Cover and simmer for 5 minutes. Then add the carrot, fennel, pepper, leek, turmeric and garlic. Mix thoroughly, then cover and simmer for a further 5 minutes.

Next, put 1 tsp of olive oil in a frying pan over a medium heat. When the pan is hot, add 4 pieces of fish

Cont'd

and cook for 2-3 minutes. Turn them over and cook for another 1-2 minutes. Place on a hot plate and cook the remaining fish fillets with the second teaspoon of olive oil.

Add the mussels and prawns to the vegetables and stock, bring to the boil and cook for 2 minutes.

Put the vegetables, prawns, mussels and broth in four bowls. Place the fish fillets on top, sprinkle with parsley, chopped tomato and a sprinkle of black pepper.

Serve.

Chicken Fajitas

These smokey fajitas combine the best of Mexican cuisine with the rich taste of the American deep south.

Serves 4　　　**Prep time 10m**　　　**Cook time 40m**

1 tbsp Worcestershire sauc
1 tsp chilli powder
1 clove garlic, minced
1 tsp hot pepper sauce
500g chicken thighs, cut into strips
1 tbsp olive oil
1 onion, sliced
1 green pepper, sliced
1/2 lemon, juice of
4 tortillas

In a medium bowl, combine the Worcestershire sauce, chilli powder, garlic and pepper sauce. Add the chicken strips and turn several times to coat them thoroughly. Then leave them to marinate for 30 minutes.

Heat the olive oil in a large frying pan and add the chicken strips to the pan. Cook for 5 minutes. Add the onion and green pepper and cook for another 3 minutes. Remove from the heat and sprinkle with lemon juice. Spread the chicken, onion and green pepper mix onto the tortillas, roll them up and serve.

Salad Recipes

Greek Salad

In this classic Greek salad recipe, tomatoes, red onion and cucumbers are dressed with olive oil and finished with crumbled feta cheese.

<u>Serves 4</u>   <u>Prep time 10m</u>   <u>Cook time 0m</u>

3 tomatoes, cut into wedges
2 cucumbers, sliced
1 red onion, thinly sliced
4 tbsp olive oil
1 1/2 tsp dried oregano
200g feta cheese, crumbled
50g olives, pitted
Salt and pepper

In a salad bowl, mix the tomatoes, cucumber and onion. Sprinkle the mixture with salt and let it sit for a few minutes so that the salt can draw out the natural juices from the tomato and cucumber.

Drizzle with olive oil and sprinkle with oregano and pepper to taste. Finish by covering the salad with feta cheese and olives. Serve.

Couscous Salad

This quick and easy to prepare salad is the ideal way to use up odds and ends left over from other meals.

<u>Serves 6</u>   <u>Prep time 10m</u>   <u>Cook time 40m</u>

180g dried couscous
1 tsp vegetable stock granules
2 tomatoes, finely chopped
2cm of cucumber, finely chopped
4 spring onions, chopped
1/2 can sweetcorn, drained
2 tbsp fresh mint, chopped
1 tbsp lemon balm, chopped
1 tbsp lemon juice
1 tbsp olive oil

Prepare the couscous by placing it and the vegetable stock granules in a large bowl and covering with boiling water so that all the couscous is covered. Place a clean dry tea towel over the bowl and allow the steam to cook the couscous. After 10 minutes, fork it through to loosen the grains.

When the couscous is cool, add the other ingredients and mix well. Place in the fridge to cool for 30 minutes while all the herbs and mint flavour are absorbed by the couscous. Serve.

Quinoa Salad

A quinoa salad that's perfect for picnics, barbecues or packed lunches.

<u>Serves 6</u>   <u>Prep time 10m</u>   <u>Cook time 15m</u>

170g quinoa, rinsed
100g cherry tomatoes, halved
55g black olives, pitted and sliced
125g feta cheese, crumbled
4 tbsp roasted sunflower seeds
1 onion, finely chopped
4 tbsp fresh parsley, chopped
3 tbsp olive oil
3 tbsp lemon juice
1 tsp Dijon mustard
2cm root garlic, finely chopped

In a bowl, mix the tomatoes and onion and then put to one side. Next, in a medium saucepan, mix the quinoa with water and bring it to the boil. Let it simmer for 15 minutes before taking it off the heat to cool.

When it has, put it in a bowl together with the tomato and onion mix, the olives, feta cheese, sunflower seeds, and parsley. Toss to combine. In a separate bowl, whisk the olive oil, lemon juice, Dijon mustard and garlic to make a dressing. Pour the lemon dressing over the quinoa salad and toss. Then serve.

Thai Chicken Salad

The hot spiciness of this salad works well with the vegetables, creating a good balance of flavour and heat.

Serves 6   **Prep time 10m**   **Cook time 10m**

4 lime leaves
2 red chilli
3 garlic cloves
2cm root ginger
4 chicken breasts
1 tbsp olive oil, 1 tbsp sesame oil
1 tsp chilli powder
50ml fish sauce
3 tbsp lime juice
3 baby gem lettuces, leaves separated
1 cucumber, de-seeded and cut into strips

Blitz the lime leaves, chillies, garlic and ginger in a blender until very finely chopped. Then mince the chicken breasts into tiny pieces. Heat both oils in a pan and then add the lime and chilli mixture. Stir-fry for 1 minute and then add the minced chicken and chilli powder. Stir-fry for 4 minutes more before adding the fish sauce. Cook for another 5 minutes.

Remove from the heat and pour the lime juice over the chicken. Serve with the lettuce and cucumber.

Lemon and Feta Salad

A fresh and tasty salad that could have been designed for a summer's day. The pine nuts give it a deliciously crunchy texture.

Serves 4   **Prep time 10m**   **Cook time 5m**

250g fresh spinach
1 tbsp pine nuts
30g feta cheese
1 lemon, grated zest and juice of
1 tbsp olive oil
Black pepper

Wash the spinach, add it to a pan with a lid, and cook for 2-3 minutes. Drain off all the excess water and allow to it cool.

Cook the pine nuts in a dry pan and stir regularly for 1-2 minutes until they are just starting to brown. Then put to one side.

Spread the spinach on a plate and then crumble the feta cheese over it. Scatter the roasted pine nuts on top.

Finally, sprinkle the lemon zest over the dish and drizzle with the lemon juice and olive oil. Season with the black pepper and serve.

Squid and Pepper Salad

Found in every ocean, squid is one of the most widely available seafoods in the world, and is also one of the cheapest.

<u>Serves 6</u>   <u>Prep time 10m</u>   <u>Cook time 5m</u>

4 red peppers, thinly sliced
2 x 400g can chickpeas, rinsed and drained
1 bunch parsley, roughly chopped
1 red chilli, de-seeded and chopped
2 garlic cloves, finely chopped
4 tbsp olive oil
600g squid, sliced into rings
1 lemon, zest and juice of
Salt and pepper

Cook the peppers under the grill. Then put them in a large bowl together with the chickpeas, parsley, chilli and garlic. Mix thoroughly and put to one side.

Heat one tablespoon of olive oil in a frying pan and add the squid. Stir-fry it until cooked.

Then put the squid into the bowl that contains the peppers and other ingredients. Season everything with salt and pepper and then dress with the remaining oil, lemon juice and lemon zest. Serve.

Vietnamese Beef Salad

A light, filling and very healthy salad with tender beef and plenty of vegetables.

<u>Serves 6</u>   <u>Prep time 5m</u>   <u>Cook time 12m</u>

350g lean beef, cut into strips
1/2 tsp chilli flakes
2 cloves garlic, crushed
4cm root ginger, finely chopped
1 pepper, sliced
150g sweetcorn
300g bean sprouts
6 spring onions, finely chopped
1 tbsp olive oil
1/2 cucumber, finely chopped
1 lime, juice of
2 tsp soy sauce

Put the olive oil and the beef in a pan and cook for 4–5 minutes. Stir in the chilli flakes, garlic and ginger. Add the pepper, stir-frying for 2–3 minutes, followed by the baby sweetcorn. Stir-fry for 1 more minute. Add the bean sprouts and spring onions and fry for 2 minutes. Then remove from the heat and allow to cool.

Make the dressing by mixing the cucumber, lime juice and soy sauce in a bowl. Then add the cooled beef mixture, mix thoroughly and serve.

Fire Salad

Fajita seasoning makes this chicken salad a seriously HOT affair! It's also seriously high in nutrients.

<u>Serves 6</u>   <u>Prep time 5m</u>   <u>Cook time 20m</u>

2 chicken breast fillets
1 35g packet of Old El Paso Fajita Spice Mix
1 tbsp olive oil
1 400g can black beans, rinsed and drained
300g sweetcorn
100g salsa
300g mixed salad greens
1 onion, chopped
1 tomato, chopped

Coat the chicken with half of the fajita spice mix. Then heat the olive oil in a frying pan and cook the chicken for 8 minutes on each side. Cut it into strips and put them to one side.

In a saucepan, mix the beans, sweetcorn, salsa and the other half of the fajita seasoning. Heat over a medium heat until warm.

Then mix the salad greens, onion and tomato in a bowl and top with the chicken. Finally, dress it all with the bean and corn mixture.

Indian Summer Salad

Packed with antioxidants, this super-healthy, colourful salad counts as one of your 5-a-day.

Serves 6   **Prep time 20m**   **Cook time 0m**

3 carrots
1 bunch radishes
2 courgettes
1 small red onion
1 handful mint leaves, chopped
1 tbsp white wine vinegar
1 tsp Dijon mustard
1 tbsp mayonnaise
2 tbsp olive oil
Salt and pepper

Grate the three carrots into a bowl. Then thinly slice the radishes and courgettes and finely chop the onion. Mix all the vegetables together in the bowl with the mint leaves.

Make the dressing by putting the vinegar, mustard and mayonnaise in a bowl and whisking to a smooth creamy consistency. Then gradually whisk in the olive oil.

Add salt and pepper to taste and then drizzle the dressing over the salad.

Avocado and Sunflower Salad

A favourite summer salad! The sunflower seeds add texture and are also very nutritious.

Serves 4   **Prep time 15m**   **Cook time 0m**

1 tbsp red wine vinegar
1 tbsp balsamic vinegar
1 clove garlic, minced
1 tbsp mayonnaise
2 heads little gem lettuce
50g sunflower seeds
2 avocados - de-stoned and sliced
6 tbsp olive oil
Salt and pepper

Whisk the olive oil, red wine vinegar, balsamic vinegar, garlic and mayonnaise together to make the dressing. Season with salt and pepper to taste.

In a salad bowl, combine the lettuce and sunflower seeds. Toss with enough dressing to coat the salad thoroughly. Top with sliced avocado and serve.

Sausage Salad

A classic winter salad topped off with tasty sausage and onion.

<u>Serves 4</u>   <u>Prep time 5m</u>   <u>Cook time 8m</u>

1 tbsp olive oil
400g sausages
1 red onion, diced
1 tbsp mustard
1 tsp light muscovado sugar
16 cherry tomatoes
2 little gem lettuces
1 small avocado, de-stoned and diced
1/2 cucumber, diced
1 tbsp red wine vinegar

Heat the olive oil in a frying pan. Cut the sausages into chunks and add them to the pan together with the onion. Stir-fry for 2 minutes and then add the mustard, muscovado sugar and tomatoes. Fry for about 5 minutes, stirring, until the mixture is coated in the sweet mustard glaze.

Separate the lettuces into leaves and mix them with the avocado and cucumber. Then put the mixture onto a platter, ladle the hot sausage mixture on top and serve.

Soup Recipes

Lentil & Bacon Soup

A warming soup for the colder weather. Easy to prepare and extremely tasty.

<u>Serves 4</u>   <u>Prep time 10m</u>   <u>Cook time 50m</u>

1 tbsp olive oil
4 rashers smoked back bacon, diced
1 large onion, chopped
3 sticks celery, chopped
2 carrots, chopped
110g split red lentils
1.2 ltr water
1 tsp dried parsley
Salt and pepper

In a large saucepan, heat the olive oil and then fry the chopped bacon until done. Add the onion and fry for a further 2 minutes. Then add the celery, carrots, parsley and lentils and cook for a further minute.

Pour in the water and bring to the boil. Turn down the heat and simmer, covered, for 35-40 minutes, stirring occasionally to prevent sticking.

The soup can be served as it is (chunky) or liquidised with a blender.

Chickpea Soup

Come home to a bowl of this filling, low-fat soup. It's perfect for vegetarians as well.

Serves 4   Prep time 10m   Cook time 25m

1 tbsp olive oil
1 onion, chopped
2 celery sticks, chopped
2 tsp ground cumin
500ml vegetable stock
400g can chopped plum tomatoes
400g can chickpeas, rinsed and drained
100g broad beans
1/2 lemon, zest and juice of
1 handful coriander or parsley, chopped
1 pinch black pepper

Heat the oil in a large saucepan, then fry the onion and celery for 10 minutes until softened, stirring frequently. Add the cumin and fry for another minute.

Next, add the vegetable stock, tomatoes and chickpeas, plus a good pinch of black pepper. Simmer for 8 minutes and then add the broad beans and lemon juice. Cook for a further 2 minutes.

Season to taste, top with a sprinkling of lemon zest and chopped coriander or parsley and serve.

Chilli Bean Soup

A rich Mexican-style tomato and bean soup that makes a hearty winter supper.

<u>Serves 4</u>   <u>Prep time 5m</u>   <u>Cook time 30ms</u>

1 tbsp olive oil
1 large onion, chopped
2 cloves garlic, crushed
2 red chillies, finely chopped
1 tsp ground cumin
1 tsp ground cinnamon
2 400g cans kidney beans, drained and rinsed
1 400g can chopped tomatoes
1.2 ltr vegetable stock

Heat the oil in a saucepan, add the onion, garlic and chillies and fry for 2-3 minutes. Add the cumin and cinnamon and continue to fry for a further minute.

Then add the kidney beans, the chopped tomatoes and the vegetable stock to the pan. Bring to the boil, cover and let it simmer for 20 minutes.

Transfer the soup to a food processor, or blender, and blitz it to a smooth liquid. Finally, return it to the pan and heat until hot.

Bulgar Mushroom Soup

This soup from Eastern Europe is primarily a mushroom soup but it gets a lot of flavour from the other ingredients.

<u>Serves 6</u>   <u>Prep time 10m</u>   <u>Cook time 50m</u>

50g unsalted butter
1 onion, chopped
2 large mushrooms, chopped
2 tsp dried dill
1 tbsp paprika
1 tbsp soy sauce
500ml chicken stock
250ml milk
3 tbsp plain flour
1 tsp salt
Black pepper
2 tsp lemon juice
4 tbsp chopped parsley
125ml sour cream

Melt the butter in a large pot over a medium heat. Cook the onions in the butter for 5 minutes.

Add the mushrooms and cook for 5 more minutes.

Stir in the dill, paprika, soy sauce and chicken stock.

Cont'd

Then reduce the heat to low, cover the pot and allow it to simmer for 15 minutes.

In a bowl, whisk the milk and flour together and then pour the mix into the soup. Stir well, cover and simmer for another 15 minutes.

Finally, add the salt, black pepper, lemon juice, parsley and sour cream. Mix thoroughly, heat up for a couple of minutes and then serve.

Minestrone Soup

The perfect solution to a cold night in? A warming bowl of this chunky and delicious soup.

Serves 4   **Prep time 5m**   **Cook time 20m**

3 carrots, chopped
1 onion, chopped
4 celery sticks, chopped
1 tbsp olive oil
2 garlic cloves, crushed
2 potatoes, diced
2 tbsp tomato purée
2 ltr vegetable stock
400g can tomatoes, chopped
1/2 head cabbage, shredded

In a food processor, blitz the carrots, onion and celery into small pieces. Heat the oil in a pan, add the processed vegetables, garlic and potatoes, and then cook over a high heat for 5 minutes until everything is soft.

Stir in the tomato purée, vegetable stock and tomatoes. Bring to the boil, then turn down the heat and simmer, covered, for 10 minutes.

Finally, add the cabbage and simmer for another 2 minutes. Season to taste and serve.

Chicken Soup

This delicious and easy-to-prepare chicken soup will give your local Chinese take-away a run for its money.

<u>Serves 4</u>   <u>Prep time 10m</u>   <u>Cook time 40m</u>

800ml chicken stock
400g sweetcorn
100g chicken meat, cooked and shredded
1/2 tsp pepper
2 tbsp cornflour
125ml water
1 tbsp sesame oil
1 handful spring onions, chopped

Put the chicken stock, sweetcorn and chicken in a pan and bring to the boil. Then reduce the heat and add the pepper. Return to the boil.

In a bowl, mix the cornflour with the water. Add this mixture to the boiling soup and stir thoroughly until well mixed.

Season the soup with sesame oil, adding a few drops at a time. Now let the soup simmer on a low heat for 30 minutes.

When it is ready, garnish it with the chopped spring onions and serve.

Oriental Pumpkin Soup

Flavours of the mysterious East give this seasonal soup an added twist.

Serves 6   **Prep time 10m**   **Cook time 45m**

1kg pumpkin, chopped
4 tsp olive oil
1 onion, sliced
1 tbsp grated ginger
3 tbsp Thai red curry paste
400ml coconut milk
850ml vegetable stock
1 tsp lime juice
1 tsp sugar
1 red chilli, sliced

Heat the oven to 200°C. Put the pumpkin in a roasting tin and mix with half the oil, half the lime juice and the sugar. Roast for 30 minutes until it's tender.

In a pan, fry the onion and ginger in the remaining oil for 2-3 minutes until soft. Then add the curry paste, the roasted pumpkin, all but 3 tbsp of the coconut milk and the stock. Bring to a simmer and leave it for 5 minutes.

Then, whisk the soup with a hand blender until it is smooth. Season it with salt and pepper and the remaining lime juice. Serve drizzled with the reminder of the coconut milk and the chilli slices.

Peanut Soup

A hearty soup which gets its delicious flavour and lovely colour from a combination of red peppers, tomatoes, peanut butter, chilli pepper and brown rice.

<u>Serves 6</u>   <u>Prep time 5m</u>   <u>Cook time 65m</u>

2 tbsp olive oil
2 small onions, chopped
2 red peppers, chopped
4 cloves garlic, minced
700g jar passata
2 ltr vegetable stock
1/2 tsp black pepper
1/2 tsp chilli powder
200g crunchy peanut butter
85g uncooked brown rice

Heat the oil in a large saucepan over a medium heat. Cook the onions and peppers until tender. Stir in the garlic when nearly done.

Add the passata, vegetable stock, black pepper and chilli powder. Reduce the heat to low and simmer, uncovered, for 20 minutes.

Add the rice, cover, and simmer for another 40 minutes until the rice is tender. Finally, stir in the peanut butter until well blended. Serve.

Cauliflower Cheese Soup

Easier and quicker to make than cauliflower cheese, this soup still has that lovely flavour. It's rich, creamy and filling but reasonably low in calories.

<u>Serves 6</u>   <u>Prep time 5m</u>   <u>Cook time 40m</u>

1 onion, finely chopped
1 cauliflower, cut into florets
1 small potato, chopped
700ml vegetable stock
400ml milk
100g mature cheddar, diced
1 knob of butter

Heat the butter in a large saucepan. Put in the onion and cook until it's soft - about 5 minutes. Add the cauliflower, potato, vegetable stock and milk. Bring to the boil, then reduce the heat and leave to simmer for about 30 minutes until the cauliflower is soft and the potato is turning to mush.

Whisk the mixture in a blender or food processor until you get a creamy, thick soup. Add more milk to thin a little if necessary.

When ready to serve, top with the cheese pieces, then stir through before eating.

Oriental Prawn Soup

A quick and spicy wok-based soup means one pan, zero fuss and supper's on the table in 10 minutes.

Serves 4   **Prep time 0m**   **Cook time 10m**

1 tbsp olive oil
300g bag of stir-fry vegetables
140g shiitake mushroom, sliced
2 tbsp Thai green curry paste
400g can coconut milk
200ml vegetable or fish stock
300g straight-to-wok medium noodles
200g raw prawns
2 sprigs of parsley, chopped

Heat the olive oil in the wok, then add and stir-fry the vegetables and the mushrooms for 2-3 minutes. Remove from the wok and put to one side.

Put the curry paste into the wok and fry for 1 min.

Pour in the coconut milk and stock. Bring to the boil, drop in the noodles and prawns, then reduce the heat and simmer for 4 minutes until the prawns are cooked through. Stir in the vegetables, mushrooms and the chopped parsley.

The soup is now ready to serve.

Snacks

Cheesy Crisps

A quick, easy and much healthier take on shop-bought crisps. They taste a lot better too!

Makes 8   **Prep time 5m**   **Cook time 10m**

100g parmesan cheese, grated
100g cheddar cheese, grated
100g ground almonds
2 tbsp olive oil

Preheat the oven to 150°C. Then line a baking tray with greaseproof paper.

Place both cheeses, the almonds and the olive oil in a bowl and mix together thoroughly. When done, spoon eight dollops of the mixture into the baking tray.

Cook in the oven for about 10 minutes until they are starting to go brown at the edges. Then remove them and allow to cool.

Your cheesy crisps are now ready to eat.

Pork & Pear Sausage Rolls

An unusual variation of the ever popular sausage roll. Here, we've used a pear but any hard fruit, such as an apple, will be just as good.

<u>Makes 6</u>   <u>Prep time 15m</u>   <u>Cook time 20m</u>

1 onion, diced
1 large pear, cored and finely chopped
3 sprigs of rosemary, chopped
500g pork, minced
½ tsp mustard seeds
500g puff pastry
1 egg

Put the pork, onion, pear, rosemary and mustard seeds in a blender and blitz to a fine paste. Put to one side.

Roll out the pastry to a 1/2cm thick rectangle. Cut it in half and put a strip of the pork paste down the centre of each half.

Beat the egg in a small bowl and then brush the edges of the pastry with the egg. Roll up both strips of pastry and brush on the rest of the beaten egg. Finally, cut each strip into three rolls.

Score the top of each roll and then place them in an oven set to 200°C. Bake for about 20 minutes.

Quinoa Muffins

High in protein, these savoury muffins with quinoa and feta cheese can be eaten either hot or cold.

<u>Makes 8</u>   <u>Prep time 10m</u>   <u>Cook time 25m</u>

1 tbsp olive oil
1 small onion, chopped
1 clove of garlic, crushed
50g kale, finely chopped
3 eggs
250g quinoa, cooked
100g almonds, ground
50g feta cheese

Preheat the oven to 180°C.

Line a muffin tray with paper muffin cases and grease them with olive oil.

Beat the eggs in a bowl. Then add the onion, garlic, kale, quinoa and ground almonds. Crumble in the feta cheese, mix thoroughly and season to taste.

Spoon the mixture evenly into the muffin cases and bake for 20-25 minutes or until golden brown.

Feta Fritters

These courgette and feta fritters can be eaten as a snack, a starter or even a light meal.

<u>Serves 4</u>   <u>Prep time 5m</u>   <u>Cook time 5m</u>

3 courgettes, grated
1 lemon, grated zest of
1 red chilli, de-seeded and finely chopped
1 bunch of fresh mint, finely sliced
1 egg
25g plain flour
20g parmesan cheese
1 tsp oregano
100g feta cheese
1 tbsp olive oil

Beat the egg in a bowl and then add the courgette, flour, lemon zest, parmesan cheese, chilli, mint and oregano. Mix thoroughly and then crumble in the feta cheese and mix again.

Heat the olive oil in a frying pan and fry tablespoons of the mixture for a couple of minutes on each side until golden. Remove from the pan and serve.

Lemon Houmous

Houmous is so easy to make and beats shop-bought versions every time.

Serves 6   **Prep time 15m**   **Cook time 0m**

2 400g cans chickpeas, drained
2 garlic cloves, finely chopped
3 tbsp yogurt
3 tbsp Tahini paste
3 tbsp olive oil
2 lemons, zest and juice of
20g coriander
Salt and pepper

Put everything but the coriander into a blender, then whisk to a smooth consistency.

Remove from the blender and place in a bowl. Season the houmous with the salt and pepper and then add the coriander.

Spoon it into a serving bowl, drizzle with the olive oil and serve.

Squash Chunks

Chunky wedges of squash covered in a crispy, spicy coating of nuts and seeds. Extremely nutritious.

<u>Serves 4</u>   <u>Prep time 10m</u>   <u>Cook time 45m</u>

50g hazelnuts
1 tbsp coriander seeds
2 tbsp sesame seeds
1 tbsp ground cumin
1 large butternut squash
1 tbsp olive oil

Preheat the oven to 200°C.

Toast the hazelnuts in a frying pan over a medium heat until golden. Add the coriander and sesame seeds, and toast for 1 minute more. Set aside. When cool, place in a blender together with the ground cumin and whisk until thoroughly mixed.

Peel the butternut squash, remove the seeds and slice into chunks. Toss the chunks with the olive oil, then cover them with the nut and seed coating.

Line a baking tray with greaseproof paper and add the coated chunks in a single layer. Cook for 30-40 minutes, turning halfway through, until tender.

Chicken Satay Pieces

Keep these nutty chicken satay strips in the fridge for a healthy option when you're feeling a bit peckish.

Serves 2   **Prep time 15m**   **Cook time 10m**

2 tbsp chunky peanut butter
1 garlic clove, finely grated
1 tsp Madras curry powder
1 tbsp soy sauce
2 tsp lime juice
2 chicken breast fillets cut into thick strips
15cm cucumber, cut into fingers
Sweet chilli sauce

Preheat the oven to 200°C.

Place the peanut butter, garlic, curry powder, soy sauce and lime juice in a bowl and mix well. If necessary, add a splash of boiling water to achieve the thickish consistency necessary for coating.

Add the chicken strips to the bowl and mix thoroughly ensuring they are well coated. Then place the strips in a baking tin lined with greaseproof paper and cook in the oven for about 10 minutes.

Eat with the cucumber fingers and chilli sauce.

Salmon Mayonnaise Wraps

Packed with omega-3-rich salmon, these delicious wraps with avocado and mayonnaise are an extremely healthy low-carb, high-protein snack.

Serves 2   **Prep time 10m**   **Cook time 8m**

1 tsp olive oil
2 salmon fillets
1 avocado
½ tsp English mustard powder
1 tsp cider vinegar
1 tbsp capers
8 lettuce leaves
16 cherry tomatoes, halved

Brush the salmon fillets with some olive oil, put them into a pan and cook for 3-4 minutes on each side.

Scoop the avocado's meat into a bowl. Add the mustard powder and vinegar, then mash well so that the mixture has a smooth mayonnaise-like consistency. Stir in the capers. Spoon into two small dishes and put on serving plates with the lettuce leaves and tomatoes.

Slice the salmon and arrange on the plates. Spoon some of the 'mayonnaise' onto the lettuce leaves and top with salmon and cherry tomatoes. To eat, roll up the lettuce leaves into little wraps.

Stuffed Mushrooms

Mushrooms stuffed with blue cheese, bacon, onions and garlic make a delicious and very nutritious snack.

__Serves 4__   __Prep time 15m__   __Cook time 35m__

4 strips bacon
4 large mushrooms
1 tbsp butter
1 tsp olive oil
1 small onion, diced
100g cream cheese
100g blue cheese

Preheat the oven to 175°C.

Fry the bacon in the olive oil and put it to one side. Remove the stems from the mushrooms and chop them up. Put the caps to one side.

Put the butter in a pan with the mushroom stems and onion. Cook them for about 15 minutes, stirring frequently, until the onion stems caramelise. Then put the onion and mushroom mixture into a blender together with the bacon, cream cheese and blue cheese. Blend to a smooth consistency.

Stuff the mixture into the mushroom caps and put them in a baking tin lined with greaseproof paper. Bake in the oven for 15 minutes.

Desserts

Coconut Macaroons

This recipe does include a natural sweetener, but it can be reduced or even eliminated if desired. Either way, the macaroons are a very light yet satisfying dessert.

<u>Serves 2</u>   <u>Prep time 10m</u>   <u>Cook time 45m</u>

4 egg whites
4 tbsp honey
2 tsp vanilla extract
250g desiccated coconut
1 tbsp coconut oil
1 pinch of salt
75g dark chocolate

Preheat the oven to 160°C.

Whisk the egg whites with the salt until stiff. Then add the honey, vanilla, desiccated coconut and coconut oil, and mix with the egg whites.

Using a tablespoon, put large dollops of the macaroon mixture into a baking tin lined with greaseproof paper. Then bake them for about 15 minutes until they are just starting to turn brown. Remove from the oven.

Finally, melt the dark chocolate and then drizzle it over the cooked macaroons.

Chocolate & Peanut Squares

Chocolate and peanut butter could have been made for each other! The nuts give added crunchiness.

<u>Serves 4</u>   <u>Prep time 15m</u>   <u>Cook time 0m</u>

100g dark chocolate (cocoa content of at least 70%)
4 tbsp coconut oil
4 tbsp peanut butter
½ teaspoon vanilla extract
1 tsp ground cinnamon
4 tbsp peanuts, finely chopped
1 pinch salt

Melt the chocolate and coconut oil in a pan. Then add the salt, peanut butter, vanilla and cinnamon, and mix thoroughly.

Pour the batter into a small baking tin lined with greaseproof paper.

Let it cool for a while and then top with the chopped peanuts. Refrigerate.

When the batter is set, cut it into small squares. Store the chocolate and peanut squares in the refrigerator.

Blueberry Ice Cream

This blueberry ice cream is rich, creamy and delicious. Plus, you don't need an ice cream maker to make it!

Serves 6   **Prep time 90m**   **Cook time 0m**

150g heavy whipping cream
3 egg yolks
½ tsp vanilla
½ tsp ground cardamom
½ lemon, zest of
225g mascarpone cheese
150g blueberries

Put the cream in a bowl and whip it until soft peaks form. Put it to one side.

In a separate bowl, add the egg yolks, vanilla, lemon zest and cardamom, and beat until fluffy. Mix in the mascarpone cheese and then add the whipped cream.

Add the blueberries to the mixture and combine well. Then pour it into a lidded container and place it in the freezer.

Stir the ice cream thoroughly every fifteen minutes until it firms up. This will take about 90 minutes.

Chocolate Fudge

A creamy low-carb fudge that is great as a small, but delicious, dessert. Add extra flavours if you want to, or serve as it is.

Serves 6   **Prep time 10m**   **Cook time 35m**

100g dark chocolate (cocoa content of at least 70%)
200g heavy whipping cream
1 tsp vanilla extract
75g butter

Boil the cream and vanilla in a pan for one minute and then lower to a simmer. Leave it simmering for 30 minutes. Then add the butter and mix into a smooth batter.

Remove from the heat and add pieces of the chocolate. Stir until the chocolate has melted into the batter. Add additional flavouring at this stage if so desired.

Pour the batter into a medium size baking tin and let it cool in the refrigerator for a couple of hours. Then take it out and sprinkle cocoa powder on top. Cut the fudge into pieces and serve cold.

Pumpkin Pie

Sweet pumpkin, succulent coconut and a kiss of lemon, all enveloped in a creamy filling. What could be nicer!

<u>Serves 6</u>   <u>Prep time 10m</u>   <u>Cook time 45m</u>

1 tbsp butter
4 tbsp shredded coconut
450g pumpkin
100g heavy whipping cream
¼ tsp salt
2 tsp pumpkin pie spice
1 lemon, zest of
1 tsp baking powder
3 eggs

Dice the pumpkin into cubes and place in a pan. Add the whipping cream, butter and salt, and bring to the boil. Then reduce the heat and let it simmer for 20 minutes until the pumpkin is soft. At this point, add the rest of the ingredients, except for the eggs, and blend to a smooth purée using a blender/food processor.

Beat the eggs in a bowl and then add the pumpkin purée and mix well.

Preheat the oven to 200°C. Grease a baking dish with butter and line it with the coconut flakes. Then pour the batter into the baking dish and bake for 20 minutes.

Saffron Pannacotta

A bright yellow and extremely delicious dessert, this low-carb pannacotta is very easy to make.

<u>Serves 6</u>   <u>Prep time 10m</u>   <u>Cook time 15m</u>

½ tbsp unflavoured powdered gelatin water
300g heavy whipping cream
¼ tsp vanilla extract
1 pinch saffron
1 tbsp almonds, chopped
12 raspberries

Mix the gelatin with water (follow the instructions on the pack) and set aside.

In a pan, boil the cream, vanilla and saffron. Lower the heat and allow to simmer for 10 minutes.

Remove the pan from the heat and add the gelatin. Stir until completely dissolved.

Pour the pannacotta mixture into 6 glasses. Cover the top of the glasses with plastic wrap and put them in the refrigerator for at least 2 hours.

Toast the almonds in a dry, hot, frying pan for a few minutes and then put them on top of the glasses of pannacotta together with the raspberries. Serve.

Berry Crumble

This scrumptious dessert is low in carbs, sugar-free, gluten-free and can be made without added sweeteners.

<u>Serves 4</u>   <u>Prep time 5m</u>   <u>Cook time 15m</u>

1 tsp coconut oil
300g mixed berries
150g almonds
75g pecans
2 tbsp butter
1 tsp cinnamon
1 tsp vanilla extract
1/4 tsp salt
5-10 drops liquid stevia sweetener (optional)

To make the berry base, heat the coconut oil in a pan then add the berries and cook them for 3-5 minutes.

To make the crumble, put the almonds and pecans in a food processor. Add the butter, cinnamon, vanilla, salt and stevia (if using). Pulse for a few seconds until the mixture is chopped to a fine consistency.

Sprinkle the nut mixture on top of the berries and cook for 10 minutes in an oven preheated to 200°C. Remove from the oven and serve.

Lemon Squares

These lemon squares don't just taste delicious, they are also very healthy.

Serves 4　　　　**Prep time 5m**　　　　**Cook time 15m**

150g almond flour, ground
1/4 tsp salt
1 tbsp coconut oil, melted
2 tbsp butter, melted
1 tbsp pure vanilla extract
1 tbsp honey
4 eggs
2 tbsp lemon juice

Preheat the oven to 175°C. Then line a medium size baking tin with greaseproof paper.

To make the crust, put the almond flour, salt, coconut oil, butter and vanilla extract in a bowl and mix it all thoroughly into a dough.

Press the dough evenly into the bottom of the baking tin. Bake it for about 15 minutes until lightly brown.

While the crust is baking, prepare the topping. In a blender or food processor (or by hand with a whisk), mix the almond flour, honey, eggs and lemon juice to a smooth consistency.

Cont'd

Remove the crust from the oven and pour the topping evenly all over it. Then return it to the oven and bake for another 15 minutes until the topping is brown at edges.

Remove from the oven and let it cool. Then refrigerate for 2 hours to let it set. Cut into squares and serve.

Going Forward

You bought this book because you want to get your body into a state of good health and then, having done so, keep it that way. It's not just you either; there are quite literally millions of others all wanting to do the self-same thing.

Assuming you've read it all the way through, you are now much better placed to go out and actually do it.

Let's recap: I started out by explaining the basics of nutrition - what it actually is, how to recognise when you're nutrient deficient and the importance of taking a Metabolic Type test.

You then learned about the various nutrition myths out there - the ones to take note of and the ones to ignore. I've talked about body fat and cholesterol - essential knowledge for those who want to be healthy.

As being healthy requires our bodies to be free of this body fat, I then explained the pros and cons of the most popular diets.

Another essential requirement for good health is eating good food - it's not just about weight control. To this end, a considerable portion of the book has been devoted to detailing the foods you should be eating and the ones to leave alone.

I've also taken a hard look at the processed food industry and explained just how pernicious it really is. Again, knowing how this industry operates is essential knowledge for anyone who wants to lose weight and/ or achieve good health.

So, you now have all the information you need. Waste no time in putting it to good use. The longer you leave it, the harder it gets. You may even leave it too late!

You don't need a dietician and you don't need weight-loss surgery. Just put your mind to it. Lose the excess weight, exercise and eat proper food - the foods I recommend in this book. If you do, you'll have a much healthier, longer and, almost certainly, happier life.

Nutritional Value of Fresh Fruit

	Calories	Fiber	Fat	Protein	Carbs
Apple - 1 medium	95	4.5g	0.5g	0.5g	25g
Apricot - 1 medium	14	0.5g	0g	0.5g	3g
Banana - 1 medium	105	3g	0.5g	1.5g	27g
Blackberry - 1 cup	62	7.5g	0.5g	2g	14g
Blueberry - 1 cup	83	3.5g	0.5g	1g	21g
Cherry - 1 cup	74	2.5g	0g	1g	19g
Coconut meat - 1 cup	283	7g	27g	2.5g	12g
Cranberry - 1 cup	60	4g	0g	0g	10g
Dates - 1 cup	495	15g	0g	4g	133g
Elderberry - 1 cup	106	10g	0.5g	1g	27g
Figs - 1 cup	492	20g	2g	6g	127g
Grapes - 1 cup	110	1g	0g	1g	27g
Grapefruit - 1 medium	82	3g	0g	1.5g	20g
Guava - 1 medium	61	5g	1g	2.5g	13g
Kiwi - 1 medium	42	2g	0.5g	1g	10g
Lemon - 1 medium	17	1.5g	0g	0.5g	5.5g
Lime - 1 medium	20	2g	0g	0.5g	7g
Mango - 1 medium	145	3.5g	0.5g	1g	35g
Mulberry - 1 cup	60	2.5g	0.5g	2g	14g
Orange - 1 medium	62	3g	0g	1g	15g
Papaya - 1 cup	60	2.5g	0.5g	0.5g	16g
Passion Fruit - 1 med	5	0.5g	0.5g	0.5g	1g
Peach - 1 medium	38	1.5g	0g	1g	9g
Pear - 1 medium	96	5g	0g	0.5g	25g
Plum - 1 medium	20	0.5g	0g	0.5g	5g
Pineapple - 1 cup	82	2.5g	0g	1g	21g
Pomegranate - 1 med	100	1g	0.5g	1g	26g
Raspberry - 1 cup	64	8g	1g	1.5g	15g
Rhubarb - 1 cup	26	2g	0g	1g	5.5g
Strawberry - 1 cup	49	3g	0.5g	1g	12g
Watermelon - 1 cup	45	0.5g	0g	1g	11g

Nutritional Value of Dried Fruit

	Calories	Fiber	Fat	Protein	Carbs
Apple - 1 cup	240	6g	0g	1g	50g
Apricots - 1 cup	310	9.5g	0.5g	4.5g	82g
Cranberries - 1 cup	520	8g	0g	0g	136g
Dates - 1 cup	493	15g	0g	4g	133g
Figs - 1 cup	490	20g	2g	6g	127g
Goji Berries - 1 cup	300	2g	3g	18g	60g
Prunes - 1 cup	408	12g	0.5g	3.5g	109g
Raisins - 1 cup	436	5g	1g	4g	115g
Sultanas - 1 cup	656	4.5g	0g	4.5g	154g

Nutritional Value of Fruit Juices

	Calories	Fiber	Fat	Protein	Carbs
Apple - 1 cup	117	0g	0.5g	0g	29g
Beetroot - 1 cup	96	0g	0g	3g	21g
Carrot - 1 cup	80	0g	0g	2g	17g
Cranberry - 1 cup	110	0g	0g	0g	28g
Grapefruit - 1 cup	96	0g	0g	1g	23g
Lemon - 1 tablespoon	3	0g	0g	0g	1g
Lime - 1 tablespoon	5	0g	0g	0g	1.5g
Orange - 1 cup	112	0.5g	0.5g	1.5g	26g
Pineapple - 1 cup	120	0g	0g	0g	31g
Pomegranate - 1 cup	100	0g	0g	0g	20g
Prune - 1cup	180	2.5g	0g	1.5g	45g
Tomato - 1 cup	41	1g	0g	2g	10g
Coconut water - 1 cup	46	2.5g	0.5g	1.5g	9g

Nutritional Value of Vegetables

	Calories	Fiber	Fat	Protein	Carbs
Artichoke - 1 medium	60	7g	0g	4g	13g
Asparagus - 1 cup	27	3g	0g	3g	5g
Avocado - 1 medium	289	12g	26.5g	3.5g	15g
Beetroot - 1 medium	35	2.5g	0g	1.5g	8g
Broccoli - 1 cup	31	2.5g	0.5g	2.5g	6g
Brussels Sprouts - 1 cup	38	3.5g	0.5g	3g	8g
Cabbage - 1 cup	22	2g	0g	1g	5g
Carrots - 1 medium	25	1.5g	0g	0.5g	6g
Cauliflower - 1 cup	25	2.5g	0g	2g	5.5g
Celery - 1 stalk	6	0.5g	0g	0.5g	1g
Courgette - 1 medium	40	2g	1g	3.5g	5g
Cucumber - 1 medium	24	1.5g	0.5g	1g	4.5g
Eggplant - 1 medium	21	3g	0.5g	1g	5g
Fennel - 1 medium	73	7g	0.5g	3g	17g
Ginger - 1 teaspoon	1.5	1g	0g	0g	1g
Green Beans - 1 cup	34	3.5g	0g	2g	8g
Kale - 1 cup	33	1g	1g	0.5g	7g
Lettuce - 1 cup	10	0g	0g	1g	2g
Mushrooms - 1 cup	15	1g	0g	2g	2g
Onion - 1 medium	47	2.5g	0g	1.5g	10g
Parsnip - 1 cup	100	6g	0.5g	1.5g	24g
Pepper - 1 medium	30	2g	0g	1g	8g
Potato - 1 medium	164	4.5g	0g	4g	37g
Pumpkin - 1 medium	30g	0.5g	0g	1g	7.5g
Radish - 1 cup	13	1g	0g	1g	4g
Spinach - 1 cup	7	1g	0g	1g	1g
Squash - 1 cup	18	1g	0g	1.5g	4g
Sweet Potato - 1 med	112	4g	0g	3g	26g
Tomato - 1 medium	22	1.5g	0g	1g	5g
Turnip - 1 medium	34	2g	0g	1g	8g
Watercress - 1 cup	7	0.5g	0g	1g	0g
Zucchini - 1 medium	32	2g	0.5g	2.5g	6.5g

Nutritional Value of Nuts

	Calories	Fiber	Fat	Protein	Carbs
Almonds - 1 cup	823	17.5g	71g	30g	31g
Brazil - 1 cup	920	10g	93g	20g	17g
Cashews - 1 cup	960	4g	76g	28g	44g
Chestnuts - 1 cup	210	2g	2g	4g	44g
Coconut - 1 cup	490	14g	50g	7g	8g
Hazelnuts - 1 cup	720	8g	72g	16g	16g
Macadamia - 1 cup	961	11g	101g	10.5g	18.5g
Peanuts - 1 cup	825	12g	71g	38g	24g
Pecans - 1 cup	760	4g	80g	12g	16g
Pistachios - 1 cup	740	12g	52g	24g	36g
Walnuts - 1 cup	800	8g	80g	20g	16g

Nutritional Value of Seeds

	Calories	Fiber	Fat	Protein	Carbs
Chia - 1 tablespoon	67	5.5g	4.5g	3g	0.5g
Flax - 1 tablespoon	37	2g	2g	1.5g	2g
Hemp - 1 tablespoon	57	0.5g	4.5g	3.5g	0.5g
Linseeds - 1 tablespoon	49	2.5g	4g	1.5g	2.5g
Poppy - 1 tablespoon	47	1g	4g	1.5g	2g
Pumpkin - 1 tablespoon	56	0.5g	5g	3g	1g
Sesame - 1 tablespoon	52	1g	4.5g	1.5g	2g
Sunflower - 1 tablespoon	47	1g	4g	1.5g	2g

Nutritional Value of Pulses

	Calories	Fiber	Fat	Protein	Carbs
Blackeyed peas - 1 cup	200	8g	4g	12g	34g
Black beans - 1 cup	240	12g	1g	14g	46g
Broad beans - 1 cup	160	8g	0.5g	10g	28g
Butter beans - 1 cup	200	10g	0g	10g	38g
Chickpeas - 1 cup	210	7g	3g	11g	34g
Green Peas - 1 cup	117	7.5g	0.5g	8g	21g
Lentils - 1 cup	320	44g	0g	40g	80g
Mung beans - 1 cup	600	33g	1.5g	49g	110g
Pinto beans - 1 cup	670	30g	2.5g	41g	120g
Kidney beans - 1 cup	216	15.5g	0g	14g	43g
Soya beans - 1 cup	290	12g	14.5g	28g	10g
Split Peas - 1 cup	440	48g	0g	40g	112g

Nutritional Value of Misc

	Calories	Fiber	Fat	Protein	Carbs
Almond milk - 1 cup	60	0.5g	2.5g	0.5g	8g
Almond butter - 1 tbsp	102	0.5g	9g	3.5g	3g
Honey - 1 tbsp	70	0.5g	0g	0g	17g
Soya milk - 1 cup	132	1.5g	4.5g	8g	15.5g
Low-fat yoghurt - 1 cup	125	0g	2.5g	7g	19g
Low-fat milk - 1 cup	110	0g	2.5g	9g	13g
Protein powder - 1 tbsp	110	0g	1.5g	23g	1g
Peanut butter - 1 tbsp	94	1g	8g	4g	3g
Cinnamon - 1 teaspoon	6	1g	0g	0g	4g
Turmeric - 1 tbsp	24	1.5g	0.5g	1g	120g
Oats - 1 cup	166	4g	3.5g	6g	28g
Cod liver oil - 1 tbsp	135	0g	15g	0g	0g
Olive oil - 1 tbsp	120	0g	14g	0g	0g

Conversion Charts

Converting Liquid

US Cups	Metric	Imperial
1 cup	250 ml	8 fl oz
3/4 cup	180 ml	6 fl oz
2/3 cup	150 ml	5 fl oz
1/2 cup	120 ml	4 fl oz
1/3 cup	75 ml	2 1/2 fl oz
1/4 cup	60 ml	2 fl oz
1/8 cup	30 ml	1 fl oz
1 tablespoon	15 ml	1/2 fl oz
1 teaspoon	5 ml	1/6 fl oz

Converting Weight

US Cups	Metric	Imperial
1 cup	150 g	5 oz
3/4 cup	110 g	3 2/3 oz
2/3 cup	100 g	3 1/2 oz
1/2 cup	75 g	2 1/2 oz
1/3 cup	50 g	1 3/4 oz
1/4 cup	40 g	1 1/2 oz
1/8 cup	20 g	3/4 oz
1 tablespoon	10 g	1/3 oz
1 teaspoon	3 g	1/10 oz

Index

310

314

317

318